TEAS Review!

Test of Essential Academic Skills Study Guide and Practice Tests

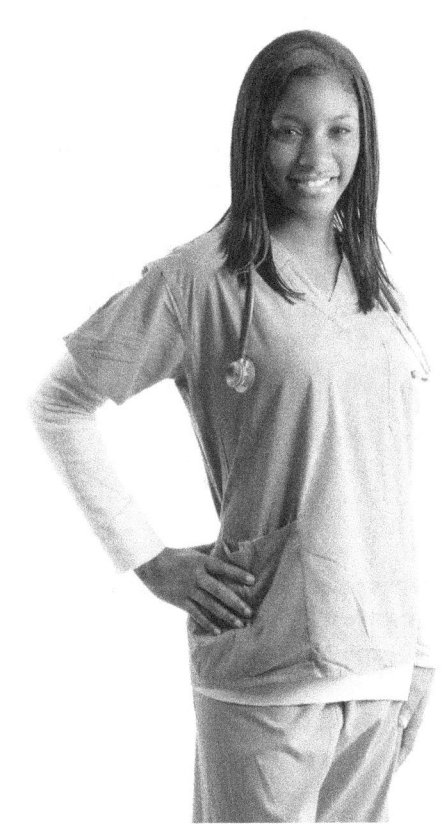

Published by

Complete TEST Preparation Inc.

Pass the TEAS!

Copyright © 2018by Complete Test Preparation Inc. ALL RIGHTS RESERVED.

No part of this book may be reproduced or transferred in any form or by any means, graphic, electronic, or mechanical, including photocopying, recording, web distribution, taping, or by any information storage retrieval system, without the written permission of the author.

Notice: Complete Test Preparation Inc. makes every reasonable effort to obtain from reliable sources accurate, complete, and timely information about the tests covered in this book. Nevertheless, changes can be made in the tests or the administration of the tests at any time and Complete Test Preparation Inc. makes no representation or warranty, either expressed or implied as to the accuracy, timeliness, or completeness of the information contained in this book. Complete Test Preparation Inc. make no representations or warranties of any kind, express or implied, about the completeness, accuracy, reliability, suitability or availability with respect to the information contained in this document for any purpose. Any reliance you place on such information is therefore strictly at your own risk.

The author(s) shall not be liable for any loss incurred as a consequence of the use and application, directly or indirectly, of any information presented in this work. Sold with the understanding, the author is not engaged in rendering professional services or advice. If advice or expert assistance is required, the services of a competent professional should be sought.

The company, product and service names used in this publication are for identification purposes only. All trademarks and registered trademarks are the property of their respective owners. Complete Test Preparation Inc. is not affiliated with any educational institution.

Complete Test Preparation Inc. is not affiliated with the makers of the TEAS V exam, Assessment Technologies Institute®, LLC, which was not involved in the production of, and does not endorse, this product.

We strongly recommend that students check with exam providers for up-to-date information regarding test content.

ISBN-13: 9781928077305

Version 7.5 March 2018

Published by
Complete Test Preparation Inc.
Victoria BC Canada

Visit us on the web at https://www.test-preparation.ca
Printed in the USA

About Complete Test Preparation Inc.

The Complete Test Preparation Team has been publishing high quality study materials since 2005. Over 1 million students visit our websites every year, and thousands of students, teachers and parents all over the world (over 100 countries) have purchased our teaching materials, curriculum, study guides and practice tests.

Complete Test Preparation is committed to providing students with the best study materials and practice tests available on the market. Members of our team combine years of teaching experience, with experienced writers and editors, all with advanced degrees.

Feedback

We welcome your feedback. Email us at feedback@test-preparation.ca with your comments and suggestions. We carefully review all suggestions and often incorporate reader suggestions into upcoming versions. As a Print on Demand Publisher, we update our products frequently.

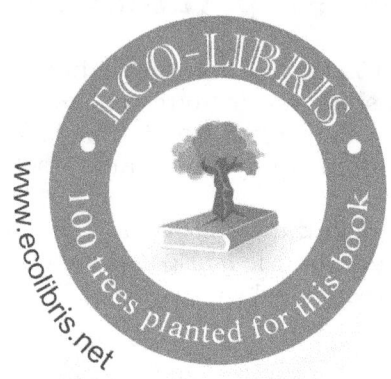

This Title is Ecologically Balanced

Through our partnership with Eco Libris, this publication is ecologically balanced. 100 trees have been planted using the highest ecological and sustainable standards in Latin America (Nicaragua, Guatemala, Panama, Belize, Honduras) and Africa (Malawi), where deforestation is a crucial problem.

Planting trees not only helps to fight climate change and conserves soil and water, but also benefits many local people, for whom these trees offer many benefits, such as improvement of crops and additional food and income, and an opportunity for a better future.

Environmental consciousness is important for the continued growth of our company. Besides eco-balancing each title, as a print on demand publisher, we only print units as orders come in, which greatly reduces excess printing and waste. This revolutionary printing technology also eliminates carbon emissions from trucks hauling boxes of books everywhere to warehouses. We also maintain a commitment to recycling any waste materials that may result from the printing process. We continue to review our manufacturing practices on an ongoing basis to ensure we are doing our part to protect and improve the environment.

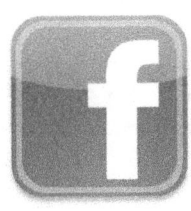 **Find us on Facebook**

www.facebook.com/CompleteTestPreparation

Contents

8 Getting Started
How this study guide is organized — 9
The TEAS® Study Plan — 9
Making a Study Schedule — 11

13 Reading
Self-Assessment — 16
Answer Key — 23
Help with Reading Comprehension — 25
Main Idea, Topic and Supporting Details — 27
Drawing Inferences And Conclusions — 30
Meaning From Context — 32

35 Mathematics
Math Self-assessment — 37
Answer Key — 42
Metric Conversion – A Quick Tutorial — 46
Fraction Tips, Tricks and Shortcuts — 48
Decimal Tips, Tricks and Shortcuts — 51
Percent Tips, Tricks and Shortcuts — 51
How to Answer Basic Math Multiple Choice — 53
How to Solve Word Problems — 56
Types of Word Problems — 58
Roman Numerals — 66

67 English and Language Usage
English and Language Usage Self-Assessment — 68
Answer Key — 76
English Grammar and Punctuation Tutorials — 78
Capitalization — 78
Colons and Semicolons — 80
Comma — 80
How to Answer English Grammar Multiple Choice - Verb Tense — 82
Common English Usage Mistakes - A Quick Review — 96
Subject Verb Agreement — 102
Help with Building your Vocabulary — 107

110 Science
Self-Assessment — 117
Answer Key — 121
Science Tutorials — 125
Scientific Method — 125
Cell Biology — 127
Chromosomes, genes, proteins, RNA and DNA — 130
Mitosis and Meiosis — 131
Phenotypes and Genotypes — 134

Heredity: Genes and Mutation	135
Heredity: Mendelian Inheritance	136
Classification	138
Basic Chemistry	140
Basic Concepts in Chemistry	141
Ecology	152
Basic Physics	156
Energy: Work and Power	160
Defining Force and Newton's Three Laws	162
Fundamental Forces: Friction	163
Fundamental Forces: Electromagnetism	164
Fundamental Forces: Gravity	166
Fundamental Forces: Strong and Weak Nuclear Forces	167
Quantum Mechanics	169
States of Matter	171

174 Human Body Science (Anatomy and Physiology)

The Circulatory System	174
The Endocrine System	183
The Integumentary System	189
The Reproductive System	194
The Respiratory System	199
The Skeletal System	204
The Nervous System	209
The Urinary System	214
The Immune System	218

223 Practice Test Questions Set 1

Practice Test 1 - Quick Reference Answer Key	263
Answer Key with Explanations	265

281 Practice Test Questions Set 2

Quick Reference Answer Key	318
Answer Key with Explanations	320

336 Conclusion

Getting Started

CONGRATULATIONS! By deciding to take the Test of Essential Academic Skills (TEAS® V) Exam, you have taken the first step toward a great future! Of course, there is no point in taking this important examination unless you intend to do your best to earn the highest grade that you possibly can. That means getting yourself organized and discovering the best approaches, methods and strategies to master the material. Yes, that will require real effort and dedication on your part, but if you are willing to focus your energy and devote the study time necessary, before you know it you will be opening that letter of acceptance to the school of your dreams.

We know that taking on a new endeavour can be scary, and it is easy to feel unsure of where to begin. That's where we come in. This study guide is designed to help you improve your test-taking skills, show you a few tricks of the trade and increase both your competency and confidence.

The Test of Essential Academic Skills Exam

Content areas for the TEAS® V are: Reading, Math, Science and English.

Reading
Paragraph Comprehension
Passage Comprehension

Mathematics
Numbers and Operations
Algebraic Applications
Data Interpretation
Measurement
Metric Conversion

Science
Human Body Science
Life Science
Earth and Physical Science
Scientific Reasoning

English and Language Usage
English Grammar and Usage
Word meaning in Context
Spelling and Punctuation
Sentence Structure

GETTING STARTED

While we seek to make our guide as comprehensive as possible, note that like all entrance exams, the TEAS® V Exam might be adjusted at some future point. New material might be added, or content that is no longer relevant or applicable might be removed. It is always a good idea to give the materials you receive when you register to take the TEAS® a careful review.

It is also important to note that not all schools use all the modules or the same version. Make sure you know which version of the TEAS and which modules your school will be using so you do not waste valuable study time studying material that is no on your school's test!

How this study guide is organized

This study guide is divided into three sections. The first section, Self-Assessments, which will help you recognize your areas of strength and weaknesses. This will be a boon when it managing your study time most efficiently; there is not much point of focusing on material you already have firmly under control. Instead, taking the self-assessments will show you where that time could be much better spent. In this area you will begin with a few questions to evaluate quickly your understanding of material that is likely to appear on the TEAS®. If you do poorly in certain areas, simply work carefully through the tutorials and then try the self-assessment again.

The second section, Tutorials, offers information in each of the content areas, as well as tactics to help you master that material. The tutorials are not intended to be a complete course, but cover general principles. If you find that you do not understand the tutorials, it is recommended that you seek out additional instruction. Note most Universities recommend students take introductory courses in Math, English and Science before taking the TEAS®.

Third, we offer two sets of practice test questions, similar to those on the TEAS® V Exam. Again, we cover all modules, so make sure to check with your school!

The TEAS® Study Plan

Now that you have made the decision to take the TEAS, it's time to get started. Before you do another thing, you will need to figure out a plan of attack. The very best study tip is to start early! The longer the time period you devote to regular study practice, the more likely you will retain the material and be able to reach it quickly. If you thought that 1x20 is the same as 2x10, guess what? It really is not, when it comes to study time. Reviewing material for just an hour per day over the course of 20 days is far better than studying for two hours a day for only 10 days. The more often you revisit a particular piece of information, the better you will know it. Not only will your grasp and understanding be better, but your ability to reach into your brain and quickly and efficiently pull out the tidbit you need, will be greatly enhanced as well.

The great Chinese scholar and philosopher Confucius believed that true knowledge could be defined as knowing what you know and what you do not know. The first step in preparing for the TEAS® Exam is to assess your strengths and weaknesses. You may already have an idea of what you know and what you do not know, but evaluating yourself using our Self-Assessment modules for each of the three areas, math, english science and reading, will clarify the details.

Making a Study Schedule

To make your study time the most productive, you will need to develop a study plan. The purpose of the plan is to organize all the bits of pieces of information in such a way that you will not feel overwhelmed. Rome was not built in a day, and learning everything you will need to know to pass the TEAS® Exam is going to take time, too. Arranging the material you need to learn into manageable chunks is the best way to go. Each study session should make you feel as though you have accomplished your goal, and your goal is simply to learn what you planned to learn during that particular session. Try to organize the content in such a way that each study session builds on previous ones. That way, you will retain the information, be better able to reach it, and review the previous bits and pieces at the same time.

Self-assessment

The Best Study Tip! The very best study tip is to start early! The longer you study regularly, the more you will retain and 'learn' the material. Studying for 1 hour per day for 20 days is far better than studying for 2 hours for 10 days.

What don't you know?

The first step is to assess your strengths and weaknesses. You may already have an idea of where your weaknesses are, or you can take our Self-assessment modules for each of the areas, math, English, science and reading.

Below is a table to assess your exam readiness in each content area. You can fill this in now, and correct if necessary after completing the self-assessments, or fill it in after you have taken the self-assessments.

Exam Readiness Assessment

Exam Component	Rate from 1 to 5
Reading	
Paragraph Comprehension	
Passage Comprehension	
English	
Grammar	
Word Meaning (Vocabulary - Meaning in Context)	
Spelling & Punctuation	
Sentence Structure	
Math	
Basic Math	
Algebra	
Data Interpretation	
Measurement	
Science	
Human Body Science (Anatomy and Physiology)	
Life Science (Biology, Ecology etc.)	
Earth and Physical Sciences	
Scientific Reasoning	

Making a Study Schedule

The key to a successful study plan is to divide the material you need to learn into manageable size and learn it, while at the same time reviewing the material that you already know.

Using the table above, any scores of 3 or below, mean you need to spend time learning, going over, and practicing this subject area. A score of 4 means you need to review the material, but you don't have to spend time re-learning. A score of 5 and you are OK with just an occasional review before the exam.

A score of 0 or 1 means you really need to work on this area and should allocate the most time and the highest priority. Some students prefer a 5-day plan and others a 10-day plan. It also depends on how much time until the exam.

Here is an example of a 5-day plan based on an example from the table above:

Basic Math: 1 Study 1 hour everyday – review on last day
Life Science: 3 Study 1 hour for 2 days then ½ hour a day, then review
Vocabulary: 4 Review every second day
Spelling: 2 Study 1 hour on the first day – then ½ hour everyday
Reading: 5 Review for ½ hour every other day
Algebra: 5 Review for ½ hour every other day
Human Body Science: 5 very confident – review a few times.

Using this example, here is a sample study plan which you can adapt to your own situation:

Day	Subject	Time
Monday		
Study	Basic Math	1 hour
Study	Spelling	1 hour
½ hour break		
Study	Life Sciences	1 hour
Review	Human Body Sciences	½ hour
Tuesday		
Study	Basic Math	1 hour
Study	Spelling	½ hour
½ hour break		
Study	Data Interpretation	½ hour
Review	Vocabulary	½ hour
Review	Grammar	½ hour
Wednesday		
Study	Basic Math	1 hour
Study	Spelling	½ hour
½ hour break		
Study	LIfe Sciences	½ hour
Review	Human Body Sciences	½ hour
Thursday		
Study	Basic Math	½ hour
Study	Spelling	½ hour
Review	Life Sciences	½ hour
½ hour break		
Review	Grammar	½ hour
Review	Vocabulary	½ hour
Friday		
Review	Basic Math	½ hour
Review	Spelling	½ hour
Review	Life Sciences	½ hour
½ hour break		
Review	Vocabulary	½ hour
Review	Grammar	½ hour

Reading

THIS SECTION CONTAINS A SELF-ASSESSMENT AND READING TUTORIAL. The tutorial is designed to familiarize general principles and the self-assessment contains general questions similar to the reading questions likely to be on the TEAS® exam, but are not intended to be identical to the exam questions. Many Universities recommend students take introductory courses before taking the TEAS® Exam. The tutorials are not designed to be a complete reading course, and it is assumed students have some familiarity with reading comprehension questions. If you do not understand parts of the tutorial, or find the tutorial difficult, it is recommended that you seek out additional instruction.

Note that these questions are for skill practice only.

Tour of the TEAS Reading Content

The TEAS® reading section has 42 questions and counts for 28% of your mark. Below is a more detailed list of the types of reading questions that generally appear on the TEAS®

- Draw logical conclusions
- Identify the author's intent, i.e. to persuade, inform, entertain, etc.
- Make predictions
- Analyze and evaluate the use of text structure to solve problems or identify sequences
- Read meters and gauges
- Identify passage types (narrative, expository, technical, persuasive, etc.)
- Follow directions
- Give the definition of a word from context
- Find specific information from different types of communication (memo, posted notice etc.)
- Find information from a table of contents or index
- Find information from a graphic (chart or similar, graphic representation)
- Identify and use scale, legends on a sample map

The questions below are not the same as you will find on the TEAS® - that would be too easy! And nobody knows what the questions will be and they change all the time. Mostly the changes consist of substituting new questions for old, but the changes can be new question formats or styles, changes to the number of questions in each section, changes to the time limits for each section and combining sections. Below are general reading questions that cover the same areas as the TEAS®. While the format and exact wording of the questions may differ slightly, and change from year to year, if you can answer the questions below, you will have no problem with the reading section of the TEAS®.

Reading Self-Assessment

The purpose of the self-assessment is:

- Identify your strengths and weaknesses.
- Develop a personalized study plan (above)
- Get accustomed to the TEAS® format
- Extra practice – the self-assessments are almost a full 3rd practice test!
- Provide a baseline score for preparing your study schedule.

Since this is a self-assessment, and depending on how confident you are with reading comprehension, timing is optional. The TEAS® has 42 reading questions. The reading section is 28% of the total score. The self-assessment has 15 questions, so allow about 15 minutes to complete this assessment.

Once complete, use the table below to assess your understanding of the content, and prepare your study schedule described in chapter 1.

80% - 100%	Excellent – you have mastered the content!
60 – 79%	Good. You have a working knowledge. Even though you can just pass this section, you may want to review the Tutorials and do some extra practice to see if you can improve your mark.
40% - 59%	Below Average. You do not understand reading comprehension problems. Review the tutorials, and retake this quiz again in a few days, before proceeding to the rest of the study guide.
Less than 40%	Poor. You have a very limited understanding of reading comprehension problems. Please review the Tutorials, and retake this quiz again in a few days, before proceeding to the rest of the study guide.

Reading Comprehension

Reading Comprehension Answer Sheet

	A	B	C	D
1	○	○	○	○
2	○	○	○	○
3	○	○	○	○
4	○	○	○	○
5	○	○	○	○
6	○	○	○	○
7	○	○	○	○
8	○	○	○	○
9	○	○	○	○
10	○	○	○	○
11	○	○	○	○
12	○	○	○	○
13	○	○	○	○
14	○	○	○	○
15	○	○	○	○
16	○	○	○	○
17	○	○	○	○

Directions: The following questions are based on several reading passages. A series of questions follow each passage. Read each passage carefully, and then answer the questions based on it. You may reread the passage as often as you wish. When you have finished answering the questions based on one passage, go right onto the next passage. Choose the best answer based on the information given and implied.

Questions 1 – 4 refer to the following passage.

Passage 1 - Who Was Anne Frank?

You may have heard mention of the word Holocaust in your History or English classes. The Holocaust took place from 1939-1945. It was an attempt by the Nazi party to purify the human race, by eliminating Jews, Gypsies, Catholics, homosexuals and others they deemed inferior to their "perfect" Aryan race. The Nazis used Concentration Camps, which were sometimes used as Death Camps, to exterminate the people they held in the camps. The saddest fact about the Holocaust was the over one million children under the age of sixteen died in a Nazi concentration camp. Just a few weeks before World War II was over, Anne Frank was one of those children to die.

Before the Nazi party began its persecution of the Jews, Anne Frank had a happy live. She was born in June of 1929. In June of 1942, for her 13th birthday, she was given a simple present which would go onto impact the lives of millions of people around the world. That gift was a small red diary that she called Kitty. This diary was to become Anne's most treasured possession when she and her family hid from the Nazi's in a secret annex above her father's office building in Amsterdam.

For 25 months, Anne, her sister Margot, her parents, another family, and an elderly Jewish dentist hid from the Nazis in this tiny annex. They were never permitted to go outside and their food and supplies were brought to them by Miep Gies and her husband, who did not believe in the Nazi persecution of the Jews. It was a very difficult life for young Anne and she used Kitty as an outlet to describe her life in hiding. After 2 years, Anne and her family were betrayed and arrested by the Nazis. To this day, nobody is exactly sure who betrayed the Frank family and the other annex residents. Anne, her mother, and her sister were separated from Otto Frank, Anne's father. Then, Anne and Margot were separated from their mother. In March of 1945, Margot Frank died of starvation in a Concentration Camp. A few days later, at the age of 15, Anne Frank died of typhus. Of all the people who hid in the Annex, only Otto Frank survived the Holocaust.

Otto Frank returned to the Annex after World War II. It was there that he found Kitty, filled with Anne's thoughts and feelings about being a persecuted Jewish girl. Otto Frank had Anne's diary published in 1947 and it has remained continuously in print ever since. Today, the diary has been published in over 55 languages and more than 24 million copies have been sold around the world. The Diary of Anne Frank tells the story of a brave young woman who tried to see the good in all people.

Reading Comprehension

1. From the context clues in the passage, what does annex mean?

    a. Attic

    b. Bedroom

    c. Basement

    d. Kitchen

2. Why do you think Anne's diary has been published in 55 languages?

    a. So everyone could understand it.

    b. So people around the world could learn more about the horrors of the Holocaust.

    c. Because Anne was Jewish but hid in Amsterdam and died in Germany.

    d. Because Otto Frank spoke many languages.

3. From the description of Anne and Margot's deaths in the passage, what can we assume typhus is?

    a. The same as starving to death.

    b. An infection the Germans gave to Anne.

    c. A disease Anne caught in the concentration camp.

    d. Poison gas used by the Germans to kill Anne.

4. In the third paragraph, what does outlet mean?

    a. A place to plug things into the wall

    b. A store where Miep bought cheap supplies for the Frank family

    c. A hiding space similar to an Annex

    d. A place where Anne could express her private thoughts.

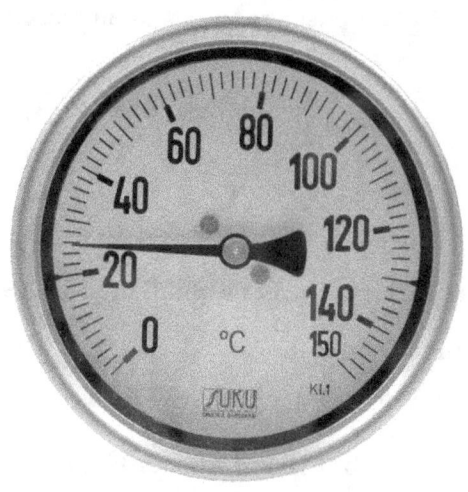

5. Consider the gauge above. What is the temperature?

    a. 26^0 C

    b. 23^0 C

    c. 22^0 C

    d. 25^0 C

Questions 6 – 9 refer to the following passage.

Passage 2 - Was Dr. Seuss A Real Doctor?

A favorite author for over 100 years, Theodor Seuss Geisel was born on March 2, 1902. Today, we celebrate the birthday of the famous "Dr. Seuss" by hosting Read Across America events throughout the March. School children around the country celebrate the "Doctor's" birthday by making hats, giving presentations and holding read aloud circles featuring some of Dr. Seuss' most famous books.

But who was Dr. Seuss? Did he go to medical school? Where was his office? You may be surprised to know that Theodor Seuss Geisel was not a medical doctor at all. He took on the nickname Dr. Seuss when he became a noted children's book author. He earned the nickname because people said his books were "as good as medicine." All these years later, his nickname has lasted and he is known as Dr. Seuss all across the world.

Think back to when you were a young child. Did you ever want to try "green eggs and ham?" Did you try to "Hop on Pop?" Do you remember learning about the environment from a creature called The Lorax? Of course, you must recall one of Seuss' most famous characters; that green Grinch who stole Christmas. These stories were all written by Dr. Seuss and featured his signature rhyming words and letters. They also featured made up words to enhance his rhyme scheme and even though many of his characters were

Reading Comprehension

made up, they sure seem real to us today.

And what of his "signature" book, The Cat in the Hat? You must remember that cat and Thing One and Thing Two from your childhood. Did you know that in the early 1950's there was a growing concern in America that children were not becoming avid readers? This was, book publishers thought, because children found books dull and uninteresting. An intelligent publisher sent Dr. Seuss a book of words that he thought all children should learn as young readers. Dr. Seuss wrote his famous story The Cat in the Hat, using those words. We can see, over the decades, just how much influence his writing has had on very young children. That is why we celebrate this doctor's birthday each March.

6. What does the word "avid" mean in the last paragraph?

  a. Good
  b. Interested
  c. Slow
  d. Fast

7. What can we infer from the statement " His books were like medicine?"

  a. His books made people feel better
  b. His books were in doctor's office waiting rooms
  c. His books took away fevers
  d. His books left a funny taste in readers' mouths.

8. Why is the publisher in the last paragraph referred to as "intelligent?"

  a. The publisher knew how to read.
  b. The publisher knew that kids did not like to read.
  c. The publisher knew Dr. Seuss would be able to create a book that sold well.
  d. The publisher knew that Dr. Seuss would be able to write a book that would get young children interested in reading.

9. The theme of this passage is

  a. Dr. Seuss was not a doctor.
  b. Dr. Seuss influenced the lives of generations of young children.
  c. Dr. Seuss wrote rhyming books.
  d. Dr. Suess' birthday is a good day to read a book.

Questions 10 - 12 refer to the following passage.

Keeping Tropical Fish

Keeping tropical fish at home or in your office used to be very popular. Today, interest has declined, but it remains as rewarding and relaxing a hobby as ever. Ask any tropical fish hobbyist, and you will hear how soothing and relaxing watching colorful fish live their lives in the aquarium. If you are considering keeping tropical fish as pets, here is a list of the basic equipment you will need.

A filter is essential for keeping your aquarium clean and your fish alive and healthy. There are different types and sizes of filters and the right size for you depends on the size of the aquarium and the level of stocking. Generally, you need a filter with a 3 to 5 times turn over rate per hour. This means that the water in the tank should go through the filter about 3 to 5 times per hour.

Most tropical fish do well in water temperatures ranging between 24^0 C and 26^0 C, though each has its own ideal water temperature. A heater with a thermostat is necessary to regulate the water temperature. Some heaters are submersible and others are not, so check carefully before you buy.

Lights are also necessary, and come in a large variety of types, strengths and sizes. A light source is necessary for plants in the tank to photosynthesize and give the tank a more attractive appearance. Even if you plan to use plastic plants, the fish still require light, although here you can use a lower strength light source.

A hood is necessary to keep dust, dirt and unwanted materials out of the tank. Sometimes the hood can also help prevent evaporation. Another requirement is aquarium gravel. This will improve the aesthetics of the aquarium and is necessary if you plan to have real plants.

10. What is the general tone of this article?

  a. Formal
  b. Informal
  c. Technical
  d. Opinion

11. Which of the following cannot be inferred?

  a. Gravel is good for aquarium plants.
  b. Fewer people have aquariums in their office than at home.
  c. The larger the tank, the larger the filter required.
  d. None of the above.

12. What evidence does the author provide to support their claim that aquarium lights are necessary?

    a. Plants require light.
    b. Fish and plants require light.
    c. The author does not provide evidence for this statement.
    d. Aquarium lights make the aquarium more attractive.

13. Which of the following is an opinion?

    a. Filter with a 3 to 5 times turn over rate per hour are required.
    b. Aquarium gravel improves the aesthetics of the aquarium.
    c. An aquarium hood keeps dust, dirt and unwanted materials out of the tank.
    d. Each type of tropical fish has its own ideal water temperature.

Questions 14 - 17 refer to the following passage.

The Civil War

The Civil War began on April 12, 1861. The first shots of the Civil War were fired in Fort Sumter, South Carolina. Note that even though more American lives were lost in the Civil War than in any other war, not one person died on that first day. The war began because eleven Southern states seceded from the Union and tried to start their own government, The Confederate States of America.

Why did the states secede? The issue of slavery was a primary cause of the Civil War. The eleven southern states relied heavily on their slaves to foster their farming and plantation lifestyles. The northern states, many of whom had already abolished slavery, did not feel that the southern states should have slaves. The north wanted to free all the slaves and President Lincoln's goal was to both end slavery and preserve the Union. He had Congress declare war on the Confederacy on April 14, 1862. For four long, blood soaked years, the North and South fought.

From 1861 to mid 1863, it seemed as if the South would win this war. However, on July 1, 1863, an epic three day battle was waged on a field in Gettysburg, Pennsylvania. Gettysburg is remembered for being the bloodiest battle in American history. At the end of the three days, the North turned the tide of the war in their favor. The North then went on to dominate the South for the remainder of the war. Most well remembered might be General Sherman's "March to The Sea," where he famously led the Union Army through Georgia and the Carolinas, burning and destroying everything in their path.
In 1865, the Union army invaded and captured the Confederate capital of Richmond Virginia. Robert E. Lee, leader of the Confederacy surrendered to General Ulysses S. Grant, leader of the Union forces, on April 9, 1865. The Civil War was over and the Union was preserved.

14. What does secede mean?

    a. To break away from

    b. To accomplish

    c. To join

    d. To lose

15. Which of the following statements summarizes a FACT from the passage?

    a. Congress declared war and then the Battle of Fort Sumter began.

    b. Congress declared war after shots were fired at Fort Sumter.

    c. President Lincoln was pro slavery

    d. President Lincoln was at Fort Sumter with Congress

16. Which event finally led the Confederacy to surrender?

    a. The battle of Gettysburg

    b. The battle of Bull Run

    c. The invasion of the confederate capital of Richmond

    d. Sherman's March to the Sea

17. What does the word abolish as used in this passage mean?

    a. To ban

    b. To polish

    c. To support

    d. To destroy

Reading Comprehension

Answer Key

1. A
We know that an annex is like an attic because the text states the annex was above Otto Frank's building.

Choice B is incorrect because an office building doesn't have bedrooms. Choice C is incorrect because a basement would be below the office building. Choice D is incorrect because there would not be a kitchen in an office building.

2. B
The diary has been published in 55 languages so people all over the world can learn about Anne. That is why the passage says it has been continuously in print.

Choice A is incorrect because it is too vague. Choice C is incorrect because it was published after Anne died and she did not write in all three languages. Choice D is incorrect because the passage does not give us any information about what languages Otto Frank spoke.

3. C
Use the process of elimination to figure this out.

Choice A cannot be the correct answer because otherwise the passage would have simply said that Anne and Margot both died of starvation. Choices B and D cannot be correct because if the Germans had done something specifically to murder Anne, the passage would have stated that directly. By the process of elimination, choice C has to be the correct answer.

4. D
We can figure this out using context clues. The paragraph is talking about Anne's diary and so, outlet in this instance is a place where Anne can pour her feelings.

Choice A is incorrect answer. That is the literal meaning of the word outlet and the passage is using the figurative meaning. Choice B is incorrect because that is the secondary literal meaning of the word outlet, as in an outlet mall. Again, we are looking for figurative meaning. Choice C is incorrect because there are no clues in the text to support that answer.

5. A
The temperature gauge is showing 26°

6. B
When someone is avid about something that means they are highly interested in the subject. The context clues are dull and boring, because they define the opposite of avid.

7. A
The author is using a simile to compare the books to medicine. Medicine is what you take when you want to feel better. They are suggesting that if a person wants to feel good, they should read Dr. Seuss' books.

Choice B is incorrect because there is no mention of a doctor's office. Choice C is incorrect because it is using the literal meaning of medicine and the author is using medicine in a figurative way. Choice D is incorrect because it makes no sense. We know not to eat books.

8. D
The publisher is described as intelligent because he knew to get in touch with a famous author to develop a book that children would be interested in reading.

Choice A is incorrect because we can assume that all book publishers must know how to read. Choice B is incorrect because it says in the article that more than one publisher was concerned about whether or not children liked to read. Choice D is incorrect because there is no mention in the article about how well The Cat in the Hat sold when it was first published.

9. B
The passage describes in detail how Dr. Seuss had a great effect on the lives of children through his writing. It names several of his books, tells how he helped children become avid readers and explains his style of writing.

Choice A is incorrect because that is just one single fact about the passage. Choice C is incorrect because that is just one single fact about the passage. Choice D is incorrect because that is just one single fact about the passage. Again, choice B is correct because it encompasses ALL the facts in the passage, not just one single fact.

10. B
The general tone is informal.

11. B
The statement, "Fewer people have aquariums in their office than at home," cannot be inferred from this article.

12. B
Light is necessary for the fish and plants.

13. B
The following statement is an opinion, " Aquarium gravel improves the aesthetics of the aquarium."

14. A
Secede means to break away from because the 11 states wanted to leave the United States and form their own country.

Choice B is incorrect because the states were not accomplishing anything. Choice C is incorrect because the states were trying to leave the USA not join it. Choice D is incorrect because the states seceded before they lost the war.

15. B
Look at the dates in the passage. The shots were fired on April 12 and Congress declared war on April 14.

Choice C is incorrect because the passage states that Lincoln was against slavery. Choice D is incorrect because it never mentions who was or was not at Fort Sumter.

16. C
The passage states that Lee surrendered to Grant after the capture of the capital of the Confederacy, which is Richmond.

Choice A is incorrect because the war continued for 2 years after Gettysburg. Choice B is incorrect because that battle is not mentioned in the passage. Choice D is incorrect because the capture of the capital occurred after the march to the sea.

17. A
When the passage said that the North had *abolished* slavery, it implies that slaves were no longer allowed in the North. In essence slavery was banned.

Choice B makes no sense relative to the context of the passage. Choice C is incorrect because we know the North was fighting slavery, not for it. Choice D is incorrect because slavery is not a tangible thing that can be destroyed. It is a practice that had to be outlawed or banned.

Help with Reading Comprehension

At first sight, reading comprehension tests look challenging especially if you are given long essays to answer only two to three questions. While reading, you might notice your attention wandering, or feeling sleepy. Do not be discouraged because there are various tactics and long range strategies that make comprehending even long, boring essays easier.

Your friends before your foes. It is always best to start with essays or passages with familiar subjects rather than those with unfamiliar ones. This approach applies the same logic as tackling easy questions before hard ones. Skip passages that do not interest you and leave them for later.

Don't use 'special' reading techniques. This is not the time for speed-reading or anything like that – just plain ordinary reading – not too slow and not too fast.

Read through the entire passage and the questions before you do anything. Many students try reading the questions first and then looking for answers in the passage thinking this approach is more efficient. What these students do not realize is that it is often hard to navigate in unfamiliar roads. If you do not familiarize yourself with the passage first, looking for answers become not only time-consuming but also dangerous because you might miss the context of the answer you are looking for. If you read the questions first you will only confuse yourself and lose valuable time.

Familiarize yourself with reading comprehension questions. If you are familiar with the common types of reading comprehension questions, you are able to take note of important parts of the passage, saving time. There are six major kinds of reading comprehension questions.

- **Main Idea** - Questions that ask for the central thought or significance of the passage.

- **Specific Details** - Questions that asks for explicitly stated ideas.

- **Drawing Inferences** - Questions that ask for a statement's intended meaning.

- **Tone or Attitude** - Questions that test your ability to sense the emotional state of the author.

- **Context Meaning** – Questions that ask for the meaning of a word depending on the context.

- **Technique** – Questions that ask for the method of organization or the writing style of the author.

Read. Read. Read. The best preparation for reading comprehension tests is always to read, read and read. If you are not used to reading lengthy passages, you will probably lose concentration. Increase your attention span by making a habit out of reading.

Reading Comprehension tests become less daunting when you have trained yourself to read and understand fast. Always remember that it is easier to understand passages you are interested in. Do not read through passages hastily. Make mental notes of ideas you may be asked.

Reading Comprehension Strategy

When facing the reading comprehension section of a standardized test, you need a strategy to be successful. You want to keep several steps in mind:

- First, make a note of the time and the number of sections. Time your work accordingly. Typically, four to five minutes per section is sufficient. Second, read the directions for each selection thoroughly before beginning (and listen well to any additional verbal instructions, as they will often clarify obscure or confusing written guidelines). You must know exactly how to do what you're about to do!

- Now you're ready to begin reading the selection. Read the passage carefully, noting significant characters or events on a scratch sheet of paper or underlining on the test sheet. Many students find making a basic list in the margins helpful. Quickly jot down or underline one-word summaries of characters, notable happenings, numbers, or key ideas. This will help you better retain information and focus wandering thoughts. Remember, however, that your main goal in doing this is to find the information that answers the questions. Even if you find the passage interesting, remember your goal and work fast but stay on track.

- Now read the question and all the choices. Now you have read the passage, have a general idea of the main ideas, and have marked the important points. Read the question and all the choices. Never choose an answer without reading them all! Questions are often designed to confuse – stay focussed and clear. Usually the answer choices will focus on one or two facts or inferences from the passage. Keep these clear in your mind.

- Search for the answer. With a very general idea of what the different choices are, go back to the passage and scan for the relevant information. Watch for big words, unusual or unique words. These make your job easier as you can scan the text for the particular word.

- Mark the Answer. Now you have the key information the question is looking for. Go back to the question, quickly scan the choices and mark the correct one.

Understand and practice the different types of standardized reading comprehension tests. See the list above for the different types. Typically, there will be several questions dealing with facts from the selection, a couple more inference questions dealing with logical consequences of those facts, and periodically an application-oriented question surfaces to force you to make connections with what you already know. Some students prefer to answer the questions as listed, and feel classifying the question and then ordering is wasting precious time. Other students prefer to answer the different types of questions in order of how easy or difficult they are. The choice is yours and do whatever works for you. If you want to try answering in order of difficulty, here is a recommended order, answer fact questions first; they're easily found within the passage. Tackle inference problems next, after re-reading the question(s) as many times as you need to. Application or 'best guess' questions usually take the longest, so, save them for last.

Use the practice tests to try out both ways of answering and see what works for you.

For more help with reading comprehension, see Multiple Choice Secrets at www.multiple-choice.ca

Main Idea, Topic and Supporting Details

Identifying the main idea, topic and supporting details in a passage can feel like an overwhelming task. The passages used for standardized tests can be boring and seem difficult. Test writers don't use interesting passages or ones that talk about things most people are familiar with. Despite these obstacles, all passages and paragraphs will have the information you need to answer the questions.

The topic of a passage or paragraph is its subject. It's the general idea and can be summed up in a word or short phrase. On some standardized tests, there is a short description of the passage if it's taken from a longer work. Make sure you read the description as it might state the topic of the passage. If not, read the passage and ask yourself, "Who or what is this about?" For example:

> Over the years, school uniforms have been hotly debated. Arguments are made that students have the right to show individuality and express themselves by choosing their own clothes. However, this brings up social and academic issues. Some kids cannot afford to wear the clothes they like and might be bullied by the "better dressed" students. With attention drawn to clothes and the individual, students will lose focus on class work and the reason they are in school. School uniforms should be mandatory.

Ask: What is this paragraph about?
Topic: school uniforms

Once you have the topic, it's easier to find the main idea. The main idea is a specific statement telling what the writer wants you to know about the topic. Writers usually state the main idea as a thesis statement. If you're looking for the main idea of a single paragraph, the main idea is called the topic sentence and will probably be the first or last sentence. If you're looking for the main idea of an entire passage, look for the thesis statement in either the first or last paragraph. The main idea is usually restated in the conclusion. To find the main idea of a passage or paragraph, follow these steps:

1. Find the topic.

2. Ask yourself, "What point is the author trying to make about the topic?"

3. Create your own sentence summarizing the author's point.
4. Look in the text for the sentence closest in meaning to yours.

Look at the example paragraph again. It's already established that the topic of the paragraph is school uniforms. What is the main idea/topic sentence?

Ask: "What point is the author trying to make about school uniforms?"

Summary: Students should wear school uniforms.

Topic sentence: School uniforms should be mandatory.
Main Idea: School uniforms should be mandatory.

Each paragraph offers supporting details to explain the main idea. The details could be facts or reasons, but they will always answer a question about the main idea. What? Where? Why? When? How? How much/many? Look at the example paragraph again. You'll notice that more than one sentence answers a question about the main idea. These are the supporting details.

Main Idea: School uniforms should be mandatory.

Ask: Why?

*Some kids cannot afford to wear clothes they like and could be bullied by the "better dressed" kids. **Supporting Detail**

*With attention drawn to clothes and the individual, Students will lose focus on class work and the reason they are in school. **Supporting Detail**

What if the author doesn't state the main idea in a topic sentence? The passage will have an implied main idea. It's not as difficult to find as it might seem. Paragraphs are always organized around ideas. To find an implied main idea, you need to know the topic and then find the relationship between the supporting details. Ask yourself, "What is the point the author is making about the relationship between the details?"

Cocoa is what makes chocolate good for you. Chocolate comes in many varieties. These delectable flavors include milk chocolate, dark chocolate, semi-sweet, and white chocolate.

Ask: What is this paragraph about?
Topic: Chocolate

Ask: What? Where? Why? When? How? How much/many?

Supporting details: Chocolate is good for you because it is made of cocoa, Chocolate is delicious, Chocolate comes in different delicious flavors

Ask: What is the relationship between the details and what is the author's point?

Main Idea: Chocolate is good because it is healthy and it tastes good.

Testing Tips for Main Idea Questions

1. Skim the questions – not the answer choices - before reading the passage.

2. Questions about main idea might use the words "theme," "generalization," or "purpose."

3. Save questions about the main idea for last. Questions can often be found in order in the passage.

3. Underline topic sentences in the passage. Most tests allow you to write in your test booklet.

4. Answer the question in your own words before looking at the answer choices. Then match your answer with an answer choice.

5. Cross out incorrect choices immediately to prevent confusion.

6. If two of the choices mean the same thing but use different words, they are BOTH incorrect.

7. If a question asks about the whole passage, cross out the choices that apply only to part of it.

8. If only part of the information is correct, that choice is incorrect.

9. An choice that is too broad is incorrect. All information needs to be backed up by the passage.

10. Choices with extreme wording are usually incorrect.

Drawing Inferences And Conclusions

Drawing inferences and making conclusions happens all the time. In fact, you probably do it every time you read—sometimes without even realizing it! For example, remember the first time you saw the movie "The Lion King." When you meet Scar for the first time, he is trapping a helpless mouse with his sharp claws preparing to eat it. When you see this action you guess that Scar is going to be one of the bad characters in the movie. Nothing appeared to tell you this. No caption came across the bottom of the screen that said "Bad Guy." No red arrow pointed to Scar and said "Evil Lion." No, you made an inference about his character based on the context clue you were given. You do the same thing when you read!

When you draw an inference or make a conclusion you are doing the same thing, you are making an educated guess based on the hints the author gives you. We call these hints "context clues." Scar trapping the innocent mouse is the context clue about Scar's character.

Usually you are making inferences and drawing conclusions the entire time you are reading. Whether you realize it or not, you are constantly making educated guesses based on context clues. Think about a time you were reading a book and something happened that you were expecting to happen. You're not psychic! Actually, you were picking up on the context clues and making inferences about what was going to happen next!

Let's try an easy example. Read the following sentences and answer the questions at the end of the passage.

> Shelly really likes to help people. She loves her job because she gets to help people every single day. However, Shelly has to work long hours and she can get called in the middle of the night for emergencies. She wears a white lab coat at work and usually she carries a stethoscope.

MATHEMATICS

What is Shelly's job?

    a. Musician

    b. Lawyer

    c. Doctor

    d. Teacher

This probably seemed easy. Drawing inferences isn't always this simple, but it is the same basic principle. How did you know Shelly was a doctor? She helps people, she works long hours, she wears a white lab coat, and she gets called in for emergencies at night. Context Clues! Nowhere in the paragraph did it say Shelly was a doctor, but you were able to draw that conclusion based on the information provided in the paragraph. This is how it's done!

There is a catch, though. Remember that when you draw inferences based on reading, you should only use the information given to you by the author. Sometimes it is easy for us to make conclusions based on knowledge that is already in our mind—but that can lead you to drawing an incorrect inference. For example, let's pretend there is a bully at your school named Brent. Now let's say you read a story and the main character's name is Brent. You could NOT infer that the character in the story is a bully just because his name is Brent. You should only use the information given to you by the author to avoid drawing the wrong conclusion.

Let's try another example.

> Social media is an extremely popular new form of connecting and communicating over the internet. Since Facebook's original launch in 2004, millions of people have joined in the social media craze. In fact, it is estimated that almost 75% of all internet users aged 18 and older use some form of social media. Facebook started at Harvard University as a way to get students connected. However, it quickly grew into a worldwide phenomenon and today, the founder of Facebook, Mark Zuckerberg has an estimated net worth of 28.5 billion dollars.
>
> Facebook is not the only social media platform, though. Other sites such as Twitter, Instagram, and Snapchat have since been invented and are quickly becoming just as popular! Many social media users actually use more than one type of social media. Furthermore, most social media sites have created mobile apps that allow people to connect via social media virtually anywhere in the world!

What is the most likely reason that other social media sites like Twitter and Instagram were created?

    a. Professors at Harvard University made it a class project.

    b. Facebook was extremely popular and other people thought they could also be successful by designing social media sites.

    c. Facebook was not connecting enough people.

    d. Mark Zuckerberg paid people to invent new social media sites because he wanted lots of competition.

Here, the correct answer is B. Facebook was extremely popular and other people thought they could also be successful by designing social media sites. How do we know this? What are the context clues? Take a look at the first paragraph. What do we know based on this paragraph? Well, one sentence refers to Facebook's original launch. This suggests that Facebook was one of the first social media sites. In addition, we know that the founder of Facebook has been extremely successful and is worth billions of dollars. From this we can infer that other people wanted to imitate Facebook's idea and become just as successful as Mark Zuckerberg.

Let's go through the other answers. If you chose A, it might be because Facebook started at Harvard University, so you drew the conclusion that all other social media sites were also started at Harvard University. However, there is no mention of class projects, professors, or students designing social media. So there doesn't seem to be enough support for choice A.

If you chose C, you might have been drawing your own conclusions based on outside information. Maybe none of your friends are on Facebook, so you made an inference that Facebook didn't connect enough people, so more sites were invented. Or maybe you think the people who connect on Facebook are too old, so you don't think Facebook connects enough people your age. This might be true, but remember inferences should be drawn from the information the author gives you!

If you chose D, you might be using the information that Mark Zuckerberg is worth over 28 billion dollars. It would be easy for him to pay others to design new sites, but remember, you need to use context clues! He is very wealthy, but that statement was giving you information about how successful Facebook was—not suggesting that he paid others to design more sites!

So remember, drawing inferences and conclusions is simply about using the information you are given to make an educated guess. You do this every single day so don't let this concept scare you. Look for the context clues, make sure they support your claim, and you'll be able to make accurate inferences and conclusions!

Meaning From Context

Often in Reading Comprehension questions, you are asked for the definition of a word, which you have to infer from the surrounding text, called "meaning in context." Here are a few examples with step-by-step solutions, and a few tips and tricks to answering meaning from context questions.

There are literally thousands and thousands of words in the English language. It is impossible for us to know what every single one of them means, but we also don't have time to Google a definition every time we read a word we don't understand! Even the smartest person in the world comes across words they don't know, but luckily we can use context clues to help us determine what things actually mean.

Reading Comprehension

Context clues are really just little hints that can help us determine the meaning of words or phrases and honestly, the easiest way to learn how to use context clues is to practice!

Let's start with a few basic examples.

> In some countries many people are not given access to schools, teachers, or books. In these countries, people might be illiterate.

You might not know what the word illiterate means, but let's use the clues in the sentence to help us. If people are not given access to schools, teachers, or books, what might happen? They probably don't learn what we learned in school so they might not know some of the things that we learned from our teachers! Illiterate actually means "unable to read or write." This makes sense based on the context clues!

Let's work through another example.

> We have so much technology today! So much technology that many people have started using tablets and computers to read ebooks instead of paper books! In fact, some of these people actually think that reading paper books is archaic!

Let's look for the context clues. Well, what do we know from this paragraph? We have a lot of technology and sometimes people read ebooks instead of paper books. From this we can draw the conclusion that ebooks are beginning to replace paper books because ebooks are newer and better. So if ebooks are newer and better, it must mean that paper books are older. Archaic actually means "very old or old-fashioned," which again we determined from the context clues.

Let's see if you can try a few on your own now.

> **Cody noticed the strawberries in his refrigerator were old and moldy, so he abstained and threw them away. What does abstained most likely mean?**
>
> a. chose not to consume
> b. washed
> c. shared
> d. cut into pieces

The correct answer here is A. The context clues told you the strawberries were old and moldy and also told you that Cody did something and then threw them away. If the strawberries were moldy, and Cody abstained, it makes sense that he didn't eat them—which is choice A.

You may have chosen answer B. If the strawberries were old and moldy, Cody could have washed them. But use ALL of the context clues. After he abstained, he threw them away. Why would Cody wash them and then throw them away? That doesn't make sense! In addition, why would he share them if they were old and moldy? Finally, I suppose Cody could have cut them into pieces, but why would he need to do that before throwing them away? It doesn't make as much sense, so choice A is the correct answer!

Let's do one more.

> Scott had a disdain for Lily ever since she lied to their boss and got him fired.
>
> a. Compassion
> b. Hate
> c. Remorse
> d. Money

The correct answer is B. Scott was fired because Lily lied. Can you imagine if this happened to you? I think you would have some pretty strong feelings just like Scott!

It's simple! By understanding the context, you can determine the meaning of even the hardest of words!

Mathematics

THIS SECTION CONTAINS A SELF-ASSESSMENT AND MATH TUTORIALS. The tutorials are designed to familiarize students with general principles and the self-assessment contains general questions similar to the mathematics questions likely to be on the TEAS® exam, but are not intended to be identical to the exam questions. Many Universities recommend students take an introductory mathematics course before taking the TEAS® Exam. The tutorials are not designed to be a complete mathematics course, and it is presumed students have some familiarity with mathematics. If you do not understand parts of the tutorial, or find the tutorial difficult, it is recommended that you seek out additional instruction.

Tour of the TEAS Mathematics Content

The TEAS Mathematics section has 30 questions and counts for 20% of your score. Below is a detailed list of the mathematics topics likely to appear on the TEAS. Make sure that you understand these topics at the very minimum.

- Convert decimals, percent, roman numerals and fractions

- Solve word problems

- Calculate percent and ratio

- Operations using fractions, percent and fractions

- Determine quantities and/or total cost from information given

- Analyze and interpret tables, graphs and charts

- Convert and estimate metric measurements

- Understand and solve simple algebra problems

The questions in the self-assessment are not the same as you will find on the TEAS® - that would be too easy! And nobody knows what the questions will be and they change all the time. Mostly, the changes consist of substituting new questions for old, but the changes also can be new question formats or styles, changes to the number of questions in each section, changes to the time limits for each section, and combining sections. While the format and exact wording of the questions may differ slightly, and change from year to year, if you can answer the questions below, you will have no problem with the Math section of the TEAS®.

Mathematics Self-Assessment

The purpose of the self-assessment is:

- Identify your strengths and weaknesses.
- Develop a personalized study plan (above)
- Get accustomed to the TEAS® format
- Extra practice – the self-assessments are almost a full 3rd practice test!
- Provide a baseline score for preparing your study schedule.

Since this is a Self-assessment, and depending on how confident you are with Math, timing yourself is optional. The TEAS® has 30 questions, to be answered in 40 minutes. This self-assessment has 30 questions, so allow 30 minutes to complete.

Once complete, use the table below to assess your understanding of the content, and prepare your study schedule described in chapter 1.

80% - 100%	Excellent – you have mastered the content!
60 – 79%	Good. You have a working knowledge. Even though you can just pass this section, you may want to review the Tutorials and do some extra practice to see if you can improve your mark.
40% - 59%	Below Average. You do not understand the mathematics content. Review the tutorials, and retake this quiz again in a few days, before proceeding to the Practice Test Questions.
Less than 40%	Poor. You have a very limited understanding of the mathematics content. Please review the Tutorials, and retake this quiz again in a few days, before proceeding to the Practice Test Questions.

MATHEMATICS

Math Self-Assessment Answer Sheet

1. A B C D   11. A B C D   21. A B C D
2. A B C D   12. A B C D   22. A B C D
3. A B C D   13. A B C D   23. A B C D
4. A B C D   14. A B C D   24. A B C D
5. A B C D   15. A B C D   25. A B C D
6. A B C D   16. A B C D   26. A B C D
7. A B C D   17. A B C D   27. A B C D
8. A B C D   18. A B C D   28. A B C D
9. A B C D   19. A B C D   29. A B C D
10. A B C D   20. A B C D   30. A B C D

1. Translate the following into an equation: six times a number plus five.

   a. 6X + 5
   b. 6(X+5)
   c. 5X + 6
   d. (6 * 5) + 5

2. Brad has agreed to buy everyone a Coke. Each drink costs $1.89, and there are 5 friends. Estimate Brad's cost.

   a. $7
   b. $8
   c. $10
   d. $12

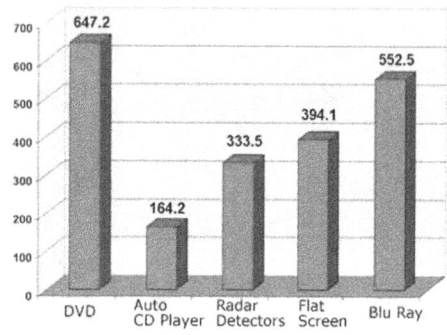

3. Consider the graph above. What is the third best-selling product?

   a. Radar Detectors
   b. Flat Screen
   c. Blu Ray
   d. Auto CD Players

4. Which two products are the closest in the number of sales?

   a. Blu Ray and Flat Screen TV
   b. Flat Screen TV and Radar Detectors
   c. Radar Detectors and Auto CD Players
   d. DVD players and Blu Ray

5. Sarah weighs 25 pounds more than Tony. If together they weigh 205 pounds, how much does Sarah weigh in kilograms? Assume 1 pound = 0.4535 kilograms.

   a. 41
   b. 48
   c. 50
   d. 52

6. A building is 15 m long and 20 m wide and 10 m high. What is the volume of the building?

   a. 45 m³
   b. 3,000 m³
   c. 1500 m³
   d. 300 m³

7. 15 is what percent of 200?

   a. 7.5%
   b. 15%
   c. 20%
   d. 17.50%

8. A boy has 5 red balls, 3 white balls and 2 yellow balls. What percent of the balls are yellow?

   a. 2%
   b. 8%
   c. 20%
   d. 12%

9. Add 10% of 300 to 50% of 20

   a. 50
   b. 40
   c. 60
   d. 45

MATHEMATICS

10. Convert 75% to a fraction.

   a. 2/100
   b. 85/100
   c. 3/4
   d. 4/7

11. Multiply 3 by 25% of 40.

   a. 75
   b. 30
   c. 68
   d. 35

12. What is 10% of 30 multiplied by 75% of 200?

   a. 450
   b. 750
   c. 20
   d. 45

13. Convert 4/20 to percent.

   a. 25%
   b. 20%
   c. 40%
   d. 30%

14. Convert 0.55 to percent.

   a. 45%
   b. 15%
   c. 75%
   d. 55%

15. A man buys an item for $420 and has a balance of $3000.00. How much did he have before his purchase?

   a. $2,580
   b. $3,420
   c. $2,420
   d. $342

16. What is the best approximate solution for 1.135 - 113.5?

   a. -110
   b. 100
   c. -90
   d. 110

17. Solve 3/4 + 2/4 + 1.2

   a. 1 1/7
   b. 2 3/4
   c. 2 9/20
   d. 3 1/4

18. The physician orders 40 mg Depo-Medrol; 80 mg/ml is on hand. How many milliliters will you give?

   a. 0.5 ml
   b. 0.80 ml
   c. 0.25 ml
   d. 0.40 ml

19. The physician orders 750 mg Tagamet liquid; 1500 mg/tsp is on hand. How many teaspoons will you give?

   a. 0.75 tsp
   b. 0.5 tsp
   c. 1 tsp
   d. 0.55 tsp

20. Convert 10 kg. to grams.

   a. 10,000 grams
   b. 1,000 grams
   c. 100 grams
   d. 10.11 grams

21. 1 gallon = _____ liter(s).

   a. 1
   b. 3.785
   c. 37.85
   d. 4.5

22. Convert 2.5 liters to milliliters.

   a. 1,050 ml.
   b. 2,500 ml.
   c. 2,050 ml.
   d. 1,500 ml.

23. Convert 210 mg. to grams.

   a. 0.21 mg.
   b. 2.1 g.
   c. 0.21 g.
   d. 2.12 g.

24. Convert 10 pounds to kilograms.

   a. 4.54 kg.
   b. 11.25 kg.
   c. 15 kg.
   d. 10.25 kg.

25. Convert 0.539 grams to milligrams.

   a. 539 g.
   b. 539 mg.
   c. 53.9 mg.
   d. 0.53 g.

26. The average weight of 13 students in a class of 15 (two were absent that day) is 42 kg. When the remaining two are weighed, the average became 42.7 kg. If one of the remaining students weighs 48 kg., how much does the other weigh?

   a. 44.7 kg.
   b. 45.6 kg.
   c. 46.5 kg.
   d. 47.4 kg.

27. The total expense of building a fence around a square-shaped field is $2000 at a rate of $5 per meter. What is the length of one side?

   a. 40 meters
   b. 80 meters
   c. 100 meters
   d. 320 meters

28. There were some oranges in a basket. By adding 8/5 of the total to the basket, the new total is 130. How many oranges were in the basket?

   a. 60
   b. 50
   c. 40
   d. 35

MATHEMATICS

29. 3 boys are asked to clean a surface that is 4 ft^2. If the surface is divided equally among the boys, how much will each clean?

    a. 1 ft 6 inches^2
    b. 14 inches^2
    c. 1 ft 2 inches^2
    d. 1 ft^2 48 inches^2

30. A person earns $25,000 per month and pays $9,000 income tax per year. The Government increased income tax by 0.5% per month and his monthly earning was increased $11,000. How much more income tax will he pay per month?

    a. $1260
    b. $1050
    c. $750
    d. $510

Math Self-assessment Answer Key

1. B
Six times a number plus five is the same as saying six times (a number plus five). Or, 6 * (a number plus five). Let X be the number so, 6(X+5).

2. C
If there are 5 friends and each drink costs $1.89, we can round up to $2 per drink and estimate the total cost at, 5 X $2 = $10. The actual cost is 5 X $1.89 = $9.45.

3. B
Flat Screen TV are the third best-selling product.

4. B
The two products that are closest in the number of sales, are Flat Screen TVs and Radar Detectors.

5. D
Let us denote Sarah's weight by "x." Then, since she weighs 25 pounds more than Tony, Tony will be x-25. They together weigh 205 pounds which means that the sum of the two representations will be equal to 205:

Sarah : x

Tony : x - 25

x + (x - 25) = 205 ... by arranging this equation we have:

x + x - 25 = 205

2x - 25 = 205 ... we add 25 to each side in order to have x term alone:

2x - 25 + 25 = 205 + 25

2x = 230

x = 230/2

x = 115 pounds → Sarah weighs 115 pounds. Since 1 pound is 0.4535 kilograms, we need to multiply 115 by 0.4535 in order to have her weight in kilograms:

x = 115 • 0.4535 = 52.1525 kilograms → this is equal to 52 when rounded to the nearest whole number.

6. B
Formula for volume of a shape is L x W x H = 15 x 20 x 10 = 3,000 m³

7. A
15/200 = X/100

MATHEMATICS

200X = (15 * 100)
1500/200 Cancel zeroes in the numerator and denominator
15/2 = 7.5%.

Notice that the questions asks, What 15 is what percent of 200? The question does *not* ask, what is 15% of 200! The answers are very different.

8. C
Total no. of balls = 10, no. of yellow balls = 2, answer = 2/10 X 100 = 20%.

9. B
10% of 300 = 30 and 50% of 20 = 10 so 30 + 10 = 40.

10. C
75% = 75/100 = 3/4

11. B
25% of 40 = 10 and 10 x 3 = 30

12. A
10% of 30 = 3 and 75% of 200 = 150, 3 X 150 = 450

13. B
4/20 X 100 = 1/5 X 100 = 20%

14. D
0.55 X 100 = 55%

15. B
(Amount Spent) $420 + $3000 (Balance) = $3,420.00

16. A
1.135 -113.5 = -112.37. Best approximate = -110

17. C
3/4 + 2/4 + 1.2, first convert the decimal to fraction, = 3/4 + 2/4 + 1 1/5 = 3/4 + 2/4 + 6/5 = (find common denominator) (15 + 10 + 24)/20 = 49/20 = 2 9/20

18. A
Set up the formula -
Dose ordered/Dose on hand X Quantity/1 = Dosage
40 mg/80 mg X 1 ML/1 = 40/80 = 0.5 mL

19. B
Set up the formula -
Dose ordered/Dose on hand X Quantity/1 = Dosage
750 mg/1500 mg X 1 tsp/1 = 750/1500 = 0.5 tsp

20. A
1kg = 1,000 g and 10 kg = 10 x 1,000 = 10,000 g

21. B
1 US gallon = 3.78541178 liters

22. B
1 liter = 1,000 milliliters, 2.5 liters = 2.5 x 1,000 = 2,500 milliliters

23. C
1,000 mg = 1 g, 210 mg = 210/1000 = 0.21 g.   Be careful of Choice A, (0.21 **mg.**) The numbers are the same but the units are different.

24. A
1 pound = 0.45 kg, 10 pounds = 4.53592, or about 4.54 kg.   When multiplying a decimal by 10, move the decimal point one place to the left.

25. B
1 g = 1,000 mg. 0.539 g = 0.539 x 1000 = 539 mg.

26. C
Total weight of 13 students with average 42 will be = 42•13 = 546 kg.

The total weight of the remaining 2 will be found by subtracting the total weight of 13 students from the total weight of 15 students: 640.5 - 546 = 94.5 kg.

94.5 = the total weight of two students. One of these students weigh 48 kg, so;

The weight of the other will be = 94.5 – 48 = 46.5 kg

27. C
Total expense is $2000 and we are informed that $5 is spent per meter. Combining these two information, we know that the total length of the fence is 2000/5 = 400 meters.

The fence is built around a square shaped field. If one side of the square is "a," the perimeter of the square is "4a." Here, the perimeter is equal to 400 meters. So,

400 = 4a

100 = a → this means that one side of the square is equal to 100 meters

28. B
Let the number of oranges in the basket before additions = x
Then: X + 8x/5 = 130
5x + 8x = 650
650 = 13x
X = 50

29. D
1 foot is equal to 12 inches. So 1 ft^2 = 12•12 in^2

4 ft^2 = 4•12•12 in^2 = 576 in^2

MATHEMATICS

This amount of surface area is divided equally among 3 boys.

Each boy will clean 576/3 = 192 in²

192 in² = 144 in² + 48 in²; 144 in² = 1 ft²

So, each boy will clean 1 ft² and 48 in²

30. D

The income tax per year is $9,000. So, the income tax per month is 9,000/12 = $750.

This person earns $25,000 per month and pays $750 income tax. We need to find the rate of the income tax:

Tax rate: 750•100/25,000 = 3%

Government increased this rate by 0.5% so it became 3.5%.

The income of the person per month is increased $11,000 so it became: $25,000 + $11,000 = $36,000.

The new monthly income tax is: 36,000•3.5/100 = $1260.

Amount of increase in tax per month is: $1260 - $750 = $510.

Metric Conversion – A Quick Tutorial

Conversion between metric and standard units can be tricky since the units of distance, volume, area and temperature can seem arbitrary when compared to each other. Although the metric system (using SI units) is the standard system of measure in most parts of the world, many countries still use at least some of their traditional units of measure. In North America those units come from the old British system.

Distance

When measuring distance, the relation between metric and standard units looks like this:

0.039 in	1 millimeter	1 inch	25.4 mm
3.28 ft	1 meter	1 foot	.305 m
0.621 mi	1 kilometer	1 mile	1.61 km

Here, you can see that 1 millimeter is equal to .039 inches and 1 inch equals 25.4 millimeters.

Area

When measuring area, the relation between metric and standard looks like this:

.0016 in^2	1 square millimeter	1 square inch	645.2 mm^2
10.764 ft^2	1 square meter	1 square foot	.093 m^2
.386 mi^2	1 square kilometer	1 square mile	2.59 km^2
2.47 ac	hectare	1 acre	.405 ha

Volume

Similarly, when measuring volume, the relation between metric and standard units looks like this:

3034 fl oz	1 milliliter	1 fluid ounce	29.57 ml
.0264 gal	1 liter	1 gallon	3.785 L
35.314 ft^3	1 cubic meter	1 cubic foot	.028 m^3

MATHEMATICS

Weight and Mass

When measuring weight and mass, the relation between metric and standard units looks like this:

.035 oz	1 gram	1 ounce	28.35 g
2.202 lbs	1 kilogram	1 pound	.454 kg
1.103 T	1 metric ton	1 ton	.907 t

Note that in science, the metric units of grams and kilograms are always used to denote the mass of an object rather than its weight.

Temperature

In predominantly metric countries the standard unit of temperature is degrees Celsius while in countries with only limited use of the metric system, such as the United States, degrees Fahrenheit is used. The chart shows the difference between Fahrenheit and Celsius:

0° Celsius	32° Fahrenheit
10° Celsius	50° Fahrenheit
20° Celsius	68° Fahrenheit
30° Celsius	86° Fahrenheit
40° Celsius	104° Fahrenheit
50° Celsius	122° Fahrenheit
60° Celsius	140° Fahrenheit
70° Celsius	158° Fahrenheit
80° Celsius	176° Fahrenheit
90° Celsius	194° Fahrenheit
100° Celsius	212° Fahrenheit

As you can see 0° C is freezing while 32° F is freezing. Similarity, 100° C is boiling compared with 212° F. To convert from Celsius to Fahrenheit you need to multiply the temperature in Celsius by 1.8, and then add 32 to it. (x° F = (y° C*1.8) + 32) To convert from Fahrenheit to Celsius you do the opposite. Subtract 32 from the temperature, then divide by 1.8. (x° C = (y° -32) / 1.8)

Fraction Tips, Tricks and Shortcuts

When you are writing an exam, time is precious, and anything you can do to answer faster is a real advantage. Here are some ideas, shortcuts, tips and tricks that can speed up answering fractions problems.

Remember that a fraction is just a number which names a portion of something. For instance, instead of having a whole pie, a fraction says you have a part of a pie--such as a half of one or a fourth of one.

Two digits make up a fraction. The digit on top is known as the numerator. The digit on the bottom is known as the denominator. To remember which is which, just remember that "denominator" and "down" both start with a "d." And the "downstairs" number is the denominator. So for instance, in ½, the numerator is the 1 and the denominator (or "downstairs") number is the 2.

- It's easy to add two fractions if they have the same denominator. Just add the digits on top, and leave the bottom one the same: 1/10 + 6/10 = 7/10.

- It's the same with subtracting fractions with the same denominator: 7/10 - 6/10 = 1/10.

- Adding and subtracting fractions with different denominators is a little more complicated. First, you have to get the problem so that they do have the same denominators. The easiest way to do this is to multiply the denominators: For 2/5 + 1/2 multiply 5 by 2. Now you have a denominator of 10. But now you have to change the top numbers too. Since you multiplied the 5 in 2/5 by 2, you also multiply the 2 by 2, to get 4. So the first number is now 4/10. Since you multiplied the second number times 5, you also multiply its top number by 5, to get a final fraction of 5/10. Now you can add 5 and 4 together to get a final sum of 9/10.

- Sometimes you'll be asked to reduce a fraction to its simplest form. This means getting it to where the only common factor of the numerator and denominator is 1. Think of it this way: Numerators and denominators are brothers that must be treated the same. If you do something to one, you must do it to the other, or it's just not fair. For instance, if you divide your numerator by 2, then you should also divide the denominator by the same. Let's take an example: The fraction 2/10. This is not reduced to its simplest terms because there is a number that will divide evenly into both: the number 2. We want to make it so that the only number that will divide evenly into both is 1. What can we divide into 2 to get 1? The number 2, of course! Now to be "fair," we have to do the same thing to the denominator: Divide 2 into 10 and you get 5. So our new, reduced fraction is 1/5.

- In some ways, multiplying fractions is the easiest of all: Just multiply the two top numbers and then multiply the two bottom numbers. For instance, with this problem:
2/5 X 2/3 you multiply 2 by 2 and get a top number of 4; then multiply 5 by 3 and get a bottom number of 15. Your answer is 4/15.

MATHEMATICS

☐ Dividing fractions is more involved, but still not too hard. You once again multiply, but only AFTER you have turned the second fraction upside-down. To divide ⅞ by ½, turn the ½ into 2/1, then multiply the top numbers and multiply the bottom numbers: ⅞ X 2/1 gives us 14 on top and 8 on the bottom.

Converting Fractions to Decimals

There are a couple of ways to become good at converting fractions to decimals. The fastest way is to memorize some basic fraction facts. Here are fractions that you should know:

1/100 is "one hundredth," expressed as a decimal, it's .01.

1/50 is "two hundredths," expressed as a decimal, it's .02.

1/25 is "one twenty-fifths" or "four hundredths," expressed as a decimal, it's .04.

1/20 is "one twentieth" or ""five hundredths," expressed as a decimal, it's .05.

1/10 is "one tenth," expressed as a decimal, it's .1.

1/8 is "one eighth," or "one hundred twenty-five thousandths," expressed as a decimal, it's .125.

1/5 is "one fifth," or "two tenths," expressed as a decimal, it's .2.

1/4 is "one fourth" or "twenty-five hundredths," expressed as a decimal, it's .25.

1/3 is "one third" or "thirty-three hundredths," expressed as a decimal, it's .33.

1/2 is "one half" or "five tenths," expressed as a decimal, it's .5.

3/4 is "three fourths," or "seventy-five hundredths," expressed as a decimal, it's .75.

Of course, if you're no good at memorization, another good technique for converting a fraction to a decimal is to manipulate it so that the fraction's denominator is 10, 100, 1000, or some other power of 10. Here's an example: We'll start with 3/4. What is the first number in the 4 "times table" that you can multiply and get a multiple of 10? Can you multiply 4 by something to get 10? No. Can you multiply it by something to get 100? Yes! 4 X 25 is 100. So let's take that 25 and multiply it by the numerator in our fraction ¾. The numerator is 3, and 3 X 25 is 75. We'll move the decimal in 75 all the way to the left, and we find that ¾ is .75.

We'll do another one: 1/5. Again, we want to find a power of 10 that 5 goes into evenly. Will 5 go into 10? Yes! It goes 2 times. So we'll take that 2 and multiply it by our numerator, 1, and we get 2. We move the decimal in 2 all the way to the left and find that 1/5 is equal to .2.

Converting Fractions to Percent

Working with either fractions or percents can be intimidating enough. But converting from one to the other? That's a genuine nightmare for those who are not math wizards. But really, it doesn't have to be that way. Here are two ways to make it easier and faster to convert a fraction to a percent.

- First, you might remember that a fraction is nothing more than a division problem: you're dividing the bottom number into the top number. So for instance, if we start with a fraction 1/10, we are making a division problem with the 10 on the outside the bracket and the 1 on the inside. As you remember from your lessons on dividing by decimals, since 10 won't go into 1, you add a decimal and make it 10 into 1.0. 10 into 10 goes 1 time, and since it's behind the decimal, it's .1. And how do we say .1? We say "one tenth," which is exactly what we started with: 1/10. So we have a number we can work with now: .1. When we're dealing with percents, though, we're dealing strictly with hundredths (not tenths). You remember from studying decimals that adding a zero to the right of the number on the right side of the decimal does not change the value. Therefore, we can change .1 into .10 and have the same number--except it's expressed as hundredths. We have 10 hundredths. That's ten out of 100--which is just another way of saying ten percent (ten per hundred or ten out of 100). In other words .1 = .10 = 10 percent. Remember, if you're changing from a decimal to a percent, get rid of the decimal on the left and replace it with a percent mark on the right: 10%. Let's review those steps again: Divide 10 into 1. Since 10 doesn't go into 1, turn 1 into 1.0. Now divide 10 into 1.0. Since 10 goes into 10 1 time, put it there and add your decimal to make it .1. Since a percent is always "hundredths," let's change .1 into .10. Then remove the decimal on the left and replace with a percent sign on the right. The answer is 10%.

- If you're doing these conversions on a multiple-choice test, here's an idea that might be even easier and faster. Let's say you have a fraction of 1/8 and you're asked what the percent is. Since we know that "percent" means hundredths, ask yourself what number we can multiply 8 by to get 100. Since there is no number, ask what number gets us close to 100. That number is 12: 8 X 12 = 96. So it gets us a little less than 100. Now, whatever you do to the denominator, you have to do to the numerator. Let's multiply 1 X 12 and we get 12. However, since 96 is a little less than 100, we know that our answer will be a percent a little MORE than 12%. So if your possible answers on the multiple-choice test are these:

    a) 8.5%   b) 19%   c) 12.5%   d) 25%

    then we know the answer is c) 12.5%, because it's a little MORE than the 12 we got in our math problem above.

    Another way to look at this, using multiple choice strategy is you know the answer will be "about" 12. Looking at the other choices, they are all too large or too small and can be eliminated right away.

This was an easy example to demonstrate, so don't be fooled! You probably won't get such an easy question on your exam, but the principle holds just the same. By esti-

MATHEMATICS

mating your answer quickly, you can eliminate choices immediately and save precious exam time.

Decimal Tips, Tricks and Shortcuts

Converting Decimals to Fractions

One of the most important tricks for correctly converting a decimal to a fraction doesn't involve math at all. It's simply to learn to say the decimal correctly. If you say "point one" or "point 25" for .1 and .25, you'll have more trouble getting the conversion correct. However, if you know that it's called "one tenth" and "twenty-five hundredths," you're on the way to a correct conversion. That's because, if you know your fractions, you know that "one tenth" looks like this: 1/10. And "twenty-five hundredths" looks like this: 25/100.

Even if you have digits before the decimal, such as 3.4, learning how to say the word will help you with the conversion into a fraction. It's not "three point four," it's "three and four tenths." Knowing this, you know that the fraction which looks like "three and four tenths" is 3 4/10.

Of course, your conversion is not complete until you reduce the fraction to its lowest terms: It's not 25/100, but 1/4.

Converting Decimals to Percent

Changing a decimal to a percent is easy if you remember one math formula: multiply by 100. For instance, if you start with .45, you change it to a percent by simply multiplying it by 100. You then wind up with 45. Add the % sign to the end and you get 45%.

That seems easy enough, right? Think of it this way: You just take out the decimal and stick in a percent sign on the opposite sign. In other words, the decimal on the left is replaced by the % on the right.

It doesn't work that easily if the decimal is in the middle of the number. Let's use 3.7 for example. Take out the decimal in the middle and replace it with a 0 % at the end. So 3.7 converted to decimal is 370%.

Percent Tips, Tricks and Shortcuts

Percent problems are not nearly as scary as they appear, if you remember this neat trick:

Draw a cross as in:

Portion	Percent
Whole	100

In the upper left, write PORTION. In the bottom left, write WHOLE. In the top right, write PERCENT and in the bottom right, write 100. Whatever your problem is, you will leave blank the unknown, and fill in the other four parts. For example, let's suppose your problem is: Find 10% of 50. Since we know the 10% part, we put 10 in the percent corner. Since the whole number in our problem is 50, we put that in the corner marked whole. You always put 100 underneath the percent, so we leave it as is, which leaves only the top left corner blank. This is where we'll put our answer. Now simply multiply the two corner numbers that are NOT 100. Here, it's 10 X 50. That gives us 500. Now divide by the remaining corner, or 100, to get a final answer of 5. 5 is the number that goes in the upper-left corner, and is your final solution.

Another hint to remember: Percents are the same thing as hundredths in decimals. So .45 is the same as 45 hundredths or 45 percent.

Converting Percents to Decimals

Percent are simply a specific type of decimals, so it should be no surprise that converting between the two is actually simple. Here are a few tricks and shortcuts to keep in mind:

- Remember that percent literally means "per 100" or "for every 100." So when you speak of 30% you are saying 30 for every 100 or the fraction 30/100. In basic math, you learned fractions that have 10 or 100 as the denominator can easily be turned into a decimal. 30/100 is thirty hundredths, or expressed as a decimal, .30.
- Another way to look at it: To convert a percent to a decimal, simply divide the number by 100. So for instance, if the percent is 47%, divide 47 by 100. The result will be .47. Get rid of the % mark and you're done.
- Remember that the easiest way of dividing by 100 is by moving your decimal two spots to the left.

Converting Percents to Fractions

Converting percents to fractions is easy. After all, a percent is nothing except a type of fraction; it tells you what part of 100 that you're talking about. Here are some simple ideas for making the conversion from a percent to a fraction:

- If the percent is a whole number -- say 34% -- then simply write a fraction with 100 as the denominator (the bottom number). Then put the percentage itself on

Mathematics

- top. So 34% becomes 34/100.
- Now reduce as you would reduce any percent. In this case, by dividing 2 into 34 and 2 into 100, you get 17/50.
- If your percent is not a whole number -- say 3.4% --then convert it to a decimal expressed as hundredths. 3.4 is the same as 3.40 (or 3 and forty hundredths). Now ask yourself how you would express "three and forty hundredths" as a fraction. It would, of course, be 3 40/100. Reduce this and it becomes 3 2/5.

How to Answer Basic Math Multiple Choice

Math is the one section where you need to make sure that you understand the processes before you ever tackle it. That's because the time allowed on the math portion is typically so short that there's not much room for error. You have to be fast and accurate. It's imperative that before the test day arrives, you've learned all the main formulas that will be used, and then to create your own problems (and solve them).

On the actual test day, use the "Plug-Check-Check" strategy. Here's how it goes.

Read the problem, but not the answers. You'll want to work the problem first and come up with your own answers. If you did the work right, you should find your answer among the options given.

If you need help with the problem, plug actual numbers into the variables given. You'll find it easier to work with numbers than it is to work with letters. For instance, if the question asks, "If Y-4 is 2 more than Z, then Y+5 is how much more than Z?" try selecting a value for Y. Let's take 6. Your question now becomes, "If 6-4 is 2 more than Z, then 6 plus 5 is how much more than Z?" Now your answer should be easier to work with.

Check the answer choices to see if your answer matches one of those. If so, select it.

If no answer matches the one you got, re-check your math, but this time, use a different method. In math, it's common for there to be more than one way to solve a problem. As a simple example, if you multiplied 12 X 13 and did not get an answer that matches one of the answer choices, you might try adding 13 together 12 different times and see if you get a good answer.

Math Multiple Choice Strategy

The two strategies for working with basic math multiple choice are Estimation and Elimination.

Math Strategy 1 - Estimation.

Just like it sounds, try to estimate an approximate answer first. Then look at the choices.

Math Strategy 2 - Elimination.

For every question, no matter what type, eliminating obviously incorrect answers narrows the possible choices. Elimination is probably the most powerful strategy for answering multiple choice.

Here are a few basic math examples.

Solve 2/3 + 5/12

    a. 9/17

    b. 3/11

    c. 7/12

    d. 1 1/12

First estimate the answer. 2/3 is more than half and 5/12 is about half, so the answer is going to be very close to 1.

Next, Eliminate. Choice A is about 1/2 and can be eliminated, choice B is very small, less than 1/2 and can be eliminated. Choice C is close to 1/2 and can be eliminated. Leaving only choice D, which is just over 1.

Work through the solution, a common denominator is needed, a number which both 3 and 12 will divide into.
2/3 = 8/12. So, 8+5/12 = 13/12 = 1 1/12

Choice D is correct.

Solve 4/5 – 2/3

    a. 2/2

    b. 2/13

    c. 1

    d. 2/15

You can eliminate choice A, because it is 1 and since both of the numbers are close to one, the difference is going to be very small. You can eliminate choice C for the same reason.

Next, look at the denominators. Since 5 and 3 don't go into 13, you can eliminate choice B as well.

That leaves choice D.

MATHEMATICS

Checking the answer, the common denominator will be 15. So 12-10/15 = 2/15. Choice D is correct.

Fractions shortcut - Cancelling out.

In any operation with fractions, if the numerator of one fractions has a common multiple with the denominator of the other, you can cancel out. This saves time and simplifies the problem quickly, making it easier to manage.

Solve 2/15 ÷ 4/5

    a. 6/65
    b. 6/75
    c. 5/12
    d. 1/6

To divide fractions, we multiply the first fraction with the inverse of the second fraction. Therefore we have 2/15 x 5/4. The numerator of the first fraction, 2, shares a multiple with the denominator of the second fraction, 4, which is 2. These cancel out, which gives, 1/3 x 1/2 = 1/6

Cancelling Out solved the questions very quickly, but we can still use multiple choice strategies to answer.

Choice B can be eliminated because 75 is too large a denominator. Choice C can be eliminated because 5 and 15 don't go into 12.

Choice D is correct.

Decimal Multiple Choice Strategy and Shortcuts.

Multiplying decimals gives a very quick way to estimate and eliminate choices. Anytime that you multiply decimals, it is going to give an answer with the same number of decimal places as the combined operands.

So for example,

2.38 X 1.2 will produce a number with three places of decimal, which is 2.856.

Here are a few examples with step-by-step explanation:

Solve 2.06 x 1.2

    a. 24.82

    b. 2.482

    c. 24.72

    d. 2.472

This is a simple question, but even before you start calculating, you can eliminate several choices. When multiplying decimals, there will always be as many numbers behind the decimal place in the answer as the sum of the ones in the initial problem, so choices A and C can be eliminated.

The correct answer is D: 2.06 x 1.2 = 2.472

Solve 20.0 ÷ 2.5

    a. 12.05

    b. 9.25

    c. 8.3

    d. 8

First estimate the answer to be around 10, and eliminate choice A. And since it'd also be an even number, you can eliminate choices B and C, leaving only choice D.

The correct Answer is D: 20.0 ÷ 2.5 = 8

How to Solve Word Problems

Most students find math word problems difficult. Tackling word problems is much easier if you have a systematic approach which we outline below.

Here is the biggest tip for studying word problems.

Practice regularly and systematically. Sounds simple and easy right? Yes it is, and yes it really does work.

Word problems are a way of thinking and require you to translate a real world problem into mathematical terms.

Some math instructors go so far as to say that learning how to think mathematically is the main reason for teaching word problems.

So what do we mean by Practice regularly and systematically? Studying word problems and math in general requires a logical and mathematical frame of mind. The only way that you can get this is by practicing regularly, which means everyday.

It is critical that you practice word problems everyday for the 5 days before the exam as a bare minimum.

If you practice and miss a day, you have lost the mathematical frame of mind and the benefit of your previous practice is pretty much gone. Anyone who has done any number of math tests will agree – you have to practice everyday.

Everything is important. The other critical point about word problems is that all the information given in the problem has some purpose. There is no unnecessary information! Word problems are typically around 50 words in 1 to 3 sentences. If the sometimes complicated relationships are to be explained in that short an explanation, every word has to count. Make sure that you use every piece of information.

Here are 9 simple steps to solve word problems.

Step 1 – Read through the problem at least three times. The first reading should be a quick scan, and the next two readings should be done slowly to answer these important questions:

What does the problem ask? (Usually located towards the end of the problem)

What does the problem imply? (This is usually a point you were asked to remember).

Mark all information, and underline all important words or phrases.

Step 2 – Try to make a pictorial representation of the problem such as a circle and an arrow to show travel. This makes the problem a bit more real and sensible to you.

A favorite word problem is something like, 1 train leaves Station A traveling at 100 km/hr and another train leaves Station B traveling at 60 km/hr. ...

Draw a line, the two stations, and the two trains at either end. This will solidify the situation in your mind.

Step 3 – Use the information you have to make a table with a blank portion to show information you do not know.

Step 4 – Assign a single letter to represent each unknown datum in your table. You can write down the unknown that each letter represents so that you do not make the error of assigning answers for the wrong unknown, because a word problem may have multiple unknowns and you will need to create equations for each unknown.

Step 5 – Translate the English terms in the word problem into a mathematical algebraic equation. Remember that the main problem with word problems is that they are not expressed in regular math equations. Your ability to correctly identify the variables and translate the word problem into an equation determines your ability to solve the problem.

Step 6 – Check the equation to see if it looks like regular equations that you are used to seeing and whether it looks sensible. Does the equation appear to represent the information in the question? Take note that you may need to rewrite some formulas needed to solve the word problem equation. For example, word distance problems may need you rewriting the distance formula, which is Distance = Time x Rate. If the word problem requires that you solve for time you will need to use Distance/Rate and Distance/Time to solve for Rate. If you understand the distance word problem you should be able to identify the variable you need to solve for.

Step 7 – Use algebra rules to solve the derived equation. Take note that the laws of equation demands that what is done on this side of the equation has to also be done on the other side. You have to solve the equation so that the unknown ends alone on one side. Where there are multiple unknowns you will need to use elimination or substitution methods to resolve all the equations.

Step 8 – Check your final answers to see if they make sense with the information given in the problem. For example if the word problem involves a discount, the final price should be less or if a product was taxed then the final answer has to cost more.

Step 9 – Cross check your answers by placing the answer or answers in the first equation to replace the unknown or unknowns. If your answer is correct then both side of the equation must equate or equal. If your answer is not correct then you may have derived a wrong equation or solved the equation wrongly. Repeat the necessary steps to correct.

Types of Word Problems

Word problems can be classified into 12 types. Below are examples of each type with a complete solution. Some types of word problems can be solved quickly using multiple choice strategies and some cannot. Always look for ways to estimate the answer and then eliminate choices.

1. Age

A girl is 10 years older than her brother. By next year, she will be twice the age of her brother. What are their ages now?

    a. 25, 15
    b. 19, 9
    c. 21, 11
    d. 29, 19

Solution: B

We will assume that the girl's age is "a" and her brother's age is "b." This means that

based on the information in the first sentence,
$a = 10 + b$

Next year, she will be twice her brother's age, which gives, $a + 1 = 2(b+1)$

We need to solve for one unknown factor and then use the answer to solve for the other. To do this we substitute the value of "a" from the first equation into the second equation. This gives

$10+b + 1 = 2b + 2$
$11 + b = 2b + 2$
$11 - 2 = 2b - b$
$b = 9$

$9 = b$ this means that her brother is 9 years old. Solving for the girl's age in the first equation gives $a = 10 + 9$. $a = 19$ the girl is aged 19. So, the girl is aged 19 and the boy is 9

2. Distance or speed

Two boats travel down a river towards the same destination, starting at the same time. One boat is traveling at 52 km/hr, and the other boat at 43 km/hr. How far apart will they be after 40 minutes?

  a. 46.67 km
  b. 19.23 km
  c. 6.4 km
  d. 14.39 km

Solution: C

After 40 minutes, the first boat will have traveled = 52 km/hr x 40 minutes/60 minutes = 34.7 km
After 40 minutes, the second boat will have traveled = 43 km/hr x 40/60 minutes = 28.66 km
Difference between the two boats will be 34.7 km – 28.66 km = 6.04 km.

Multiple Choice Strategy

First estimate the answer. The first boat is traveling 9 km. faster than the second, for 40 minutes, which is 2/3 of an hour. 2/3 of 9 = 6, as a rough guess of the distance apart.

Choices A, B and D can be eliminated right away.

3. Ratio

The instructions in a cookbook state that 700 grams of flour must be mixed in 100 ml of water, and 0.90 grams of salt added. A cook however has just 325 grams of flour. What is the quantity of water and salt that he should use?

    a. 0.41 grams and 46.4 ml
    b. 0.45 grams and 49.3 ml
    c. 0.39 grams and 39.8 ml
    d. 0.25 grams and 40.1 ml

Solution: A

The Cookbook states 700 grams of flour, but the cook only has 325. The first step is to determine the percentage of flour he has 325/700 x 100 = 46.4%
That means that 46.4% of all other items must also be used.
46.4% of 100 = 46.4 ml of water
46.4% of 0.90 = 0.41 grams of salt.

Multiple Choice Strategy

The recipe calls for 700 grams of flour but the cook only has 325, which is just less than half, the quantity of water and salt are going to be about half.

Choices C and D can be eliminated right away. Choice B is very close so be careful. Looking closely at choice B, it is exactly half, and since 325 is slightly less than half of 700, it can't be correct.

Choice A is correct.

4. Percent

An agent received $6,685 as his commission for selling a property. If his commission was 13% of the selling price, how much was the property?

    a. $68,825
    b. $121,850
    c. $49,025
    d. $51,423

Solution: D

Let's assume that the property price is x
That means from the information given, 13% of x = 6,685
Solve for x,
x = 6685 x 100/13 = $51,423

MATHEMATICS

Multiple Choice Strategy

The commission, 13%, is just over 10%, which is easier to work with. Round up $6685 to $6700, and multiple by 10 for an approximate answer. 10 X 6700 = $67,000. You can do this in your head. Choice B is much too big and can be eliminated. Choice C is too small and can be eliminated. Choices A and D are left and good possibilities.

Do the calculations to make the final choice.

5. Sales & Profit

A store owner buys merchandise for $21,045. He transports them for $3,905 and pays his staff $1,450 to stock the merchandise on his shelves. If he does not incur further costs, how much does he need to sell the items to make $5,000 profit?

   a. $32,500
   b. $29,350
   c. $32,400
   d. $31,400

Solution: D

Total cost of the items is $21,045 + $3,905 + $1,450 = $26,400
Total cost is now $26,400 + $5000 profit = $31,400

Multiple Choice Strategy

Round off and add the numbers up in your head quickly.
21,000 + 4,000 + 1500 = 26500. Add in 5000 profit for a total of 31500.

Choice B is too small and can be eliminated. Choices C and A are too large and can be eliminated.

6. Tax/Income

A woman earns $42,000 per month and pays 5% tax on her monthly income. If the Government increases her monthly taxes by $1,500, what is her income after tax?

   a. $38,400
   b. $36,050
   c. $40,500
   d. $39, 500

Solution: A

Initial tax on income was 5/100 x 42,000 = $2,100
$1,500 was added to the tax to give $2,100 + 1,500 = $3,600
Income after tax is $42,000 - $3,600 = $38,400

7. Simple Interest Word Problems

Simple interest is one type of interest problems. There are always four variables of any simple interest equation. With simple interest, you would be given three of these variables and be asked to solve for one unknown variable. With more complex interest problems, you would have to solve for multiple variables.

The four variables of simple interest are:
P – Principal which refers to the original amount of money put in the account
I – Interest or the amount of money earned as interest
r – Rate or interest rate. This MUST ALWAYS be in decimal format and not in percentage
t – Time or the amount of time the money is kept in the account to earn interest

The formula for simple interest is I = P x r x t

Example 1

A customer deposits $1,000 in a savings account with a bank that offers 2% interest. How much interest will be earned after 4 years?

For this problem, there are 3 variables as expected.

P = $1,000
t = 4 years
r = 2%
I = ?

Before we can begin solving for I using the simple interest formula, we need to first convert the rate from percentage to decimal.

2% = 2/100 = 0.02

Now we can use the formula: I = P x r x t

I = 1,000 x 0.02 x 4 = 80
This means that the $1,000 would have earned an interest of $80 after 4 years. The total in the account after 4 years will thus be principal + interest earned, or 1,000 + 80 = $1,080

Example 2

Sandra deposits $1400 in a savings account with a bank at 5% interest. How long will she have to leave the money in the bank to earn $420 as interest to buy a second-hand car?

In this example, the given information is:
I = $420
P = $1,400

r - 5%
t - ?
As usual, first we convert the rate from percentage to decimal
5% = 5/100 = 0.05

Next, we plug in the variables we know into the simple interest formula - I = P x r x t

420 = 1,400 x 0.05 x t
420 = 70 x t
420 = 70t
t = 420/70
t = 6

Sandra will have to leave her $1,400 in the bank for 6 years to earn her an interest of $420 at a rate of 5%.

Other important simple interest formula to remember

To use this formula below, do not convert r (rate) to decimal.

P = 100 x interest/ r x t
r = 100 x interest/p x t
t = 100 x interest/ p x r

8. Averaging

The average weight of 10 books is 54 grams. 2 more books were added and the average weight became 55.4. If one of the 2 new books added weighed 62.8 g, what is the weight of the other?

    a. 44.7 g
    b. 67.4 g
    c. 62 g
    d. 52 g

Solution: C

Total weight of 10 books with average 54 grams will be=10×54=540 g
Total weight of 12 books with average 55.4 will be=55.4×12=664.8 g
So total weight of the remaining 2 will be= 664.8 – 540 = 124.8 g
If one weighs 62.8, the weight of the other will be= 124.8 g – 62.8 g = 62 g

Multiple Choice Strategy

Averaging problems can be estimated by looking at which direction the average goes. If additional items are added and the average goes up, the new items much be greater than the average. If the average goes down after new items are added, the new items must be less than the average.

Here, the average is 54 grams and 2 books are added which increases the average to 55.4, so the new books must weight more than 54 grams.
Choices A and D can be eliminated right away.

9. Probability

A bag contains 15 marbles of various colors. If 3 marbles are white, 5 are red and the rest are black, what is the probability of randomly picking out a black marble from the bag?

    a. 7/15
    b. 3/15
    c. 1/5
    d. 4/15

Solution: A

Total marbles = 15
Number of black marbles = 15 − (3 + 5) = 7
Probability of picking out a black marble = 7/15

10. Two Variables

A company paid a total of $2850 to book for 6 single rooms and 4 double rooms in a hotel for one night. Another company paid $3185 to book for 13 single rooms for one night in the same hotel. What is the cost for single and double rooms in that hotel?

    a. single= $250 and double = $345
    b. single= $254 and double = $350
    c. single = $245 and double = $305
    d. single = $245 and double = $345

Solution: D

We can determine the price of single rooms from the information given of the second company. 13 single rooms = 3185.
One single room = 3185 / 13 = 245
The first company paid for 6 single rooms at $245. 245 x 6 = $1470
Total amount paid for 4 double rooms by first company = $2850 - $1470 = $1380
Cost per double room = 1380 / 4 = $345

MATHEMATICS

11. Geometry

The length of a rectangle is 5 in. more than its width. The perimeter of the rectangle is 26 in. What is the width and length of the rectangle?

    a. width = 6 inches, Length = 9 inches
    b. width = 4 inches, Length = 9 inches
    c. width = 4 inches, Length = 5 inches
    d. width = 6 inches, Length = 11 inches

Solution: B

Formula for perimeter of a rectangle is 2(L + W)
p=26, so 2(L+W) = p
The length is 5 inches more than the width, so
2(w+5) + 2w = 26
2w + 10 + 2w = 26
2w + 2w = 26 - 10
4w = 16

W = 16/4 = 4 inches

L is 5 inches more than w, so L = 5 + 4 = 9 inches.

12. Totals and fractions

A basket contains 125 oranges, mangos and apples. If 3/5 of the fruits in the basket are mangos and only 2/5 of the mangos are ripe, how many ripe mangos are there in the basket?

    a. 30
    b. 68
    c. 55
    d. 47

Solution: A
Number of mangos in the basket is 3/5 x 125 = 75
Number of ripe mangos = 2/5 x 75 = 30

Calculating Perimeter, Area and Volume

	Circle	Triangle	Square	Rectangle
Perimeter	$2\pi r$	$a + b + c$	$4a$	$2(H + w)$
Area	πr^2	$1/2 bh$	$2a$	lw
Volume	$4/3 \pi r^3$ (Sphere)	$1/3 bh$ (pyramid)	a^3 (cube)	hwl or abc

Roman Numerals

Roman numerals are based on seven symbols:

Symbol	Value
I	1
V	5
X	10
L	50
C	100
D	500
M	1,000
Q	500,000

Numbers are formed by combining symbols together and adding the values. For example, MMVI is 1000 + 1000 + 5 + 1 = 2006. Generally, symbols are placed in order of value, starting with the largest values. When smaller values precede larger values, the smaller values are subtracted from the larger values, and the result is added to the total. For example MCMXLIV = 1000 + (1000 − 100) + (50 − 10) + (5 − 1) = 1944

English and Language Usage

THIS SECTION CONTAINS AN ENGLISH SELF-ASSESSMENT AND ENGLISH TUTORIALS. The Tutorials are designed to familiarize students with general principles and the self-assessment contains general questions similar to the English questions likely to be on the TEAS® exam, but are not intended to be identical to the exam questions. Many Universities recommend students take an introductory English course before taking the TEAS® Exam. The tutorials are not designed to be a complete English course, and it is assumed that students have some familiarity with English. If you do not understand parts of the tutorial, or find the tutorial difficult, it is recommended that you seek out additional instruction.

Note that these questions are for skill practice only.

Tour of the TEAS English Content

The TEAS® English and Language Usage section has 30 questions, which count for 20% of your score. Below is a detailed list of the topics likely to appear on the TEAS®. Make sure you understand these topics at the very minimum.

- English Grammar

- Meaning in Context (Vocabulary)

- Spelling

- Punctuation

- Capitalization

- Sentence Structure

The questions below are not the same as you will find on the TEAS® - that would be too easy! And nobody knows what the questions will be and they change all the time. Mostly, the changes consist of substituting new questions for old, but the changes also can be new question formats or styles, changes to the number of questions in each section, changes to the time limits for each section, and combining sections. While the format and exact wording of the questions may differ slightly, and change from year to year, if you can answer the questions below, you will have no problem with the English section of the TEAS® V.

English and Language Usage Self-Assessment

The purpose of the self-assessment is:

- Identify your strengths and weaknesses.
- Develop a personalized study plan (above)
- Get accustomed to the TEAS® format
- Extra practice – the self-assessment is a 3rd test!
- Provide a baseline score for preparing your study schedule.

Since this is a self-assessment, and depending on how confident you are with English grammar, timing yourself is optional. The TEAS® English and language usage section has 30 questions which must be answered in 40 minutes. The self-assessment has 30 questions, so allow 40 minutes to complete this assessment.

Once complete, use the table below to assess your understanding of the content and prepare your study schedule described in chapter 1.

80% - 100%	Excellent – you have mastered the content!
60 – 79%	Good. You have a working knowledge. Even though you can just pass this section, you may want to review the Tutorials and do some extra practice to see if you can improve your mark.
40% - 59%	Below Average. You do not understand the English content. Review the tutorials, and retake this quiz again in a few days, before proceeding to the practice test questions.
Less than 40%	Poor. You have a very limited understanding. Please review the Tutorials, and retake this quiz again in a few days, before proceeding to the practice test questions.

English and Language Usage

English Self-Assessment Answer Sheet

1. A B C D
2. A B C D
3. A B C D
4. A B C D
5. A B C D
6. A B C D
7. A B C D
8. A B C D
9. A B C D
10. A B C D

11. A B C D
12. A B C D
13. A B C D
14. A B C D
15. A B C D
16. A B C D
17. A B C D
18. A B C D
19. A B C D
20. A B C D

21. A B C D
22. A B C D
23. A B C D
24. A B C D
25. A B C D
26. A B C D
27. A B C D
28. A B C D
29. A B C D
30. A B C D

Select the word that best fits the given sentence.

1. He didn't realize how serious the crime was. It wasn't simply a misdemeanor, but rather a _____.

    a. Felony
    b. Trespass
    c. Infraction
    d. None of the Above

2. Choose the correct sentence.

    a. Does the sun set in the East or West?
    b. Does the sun set in the east or the west?
    c. Does the Sun set in the east or west?
    d. None of the Above.

3. Their new house is like a castle. I have never seen such a _____ home.

    a. Palace
    b. Palatial
    c. Meagre
    d. Humble

4. Fill in the blank.

She never does anything like that, so I doubt that she will do it herself. I am sure she will get one of her _____ to do it.

    a. Superiors
    b. Acquaintances
    c. Underlings
    d. None of the Above

5. He went to the store after school.

What is the subject of this sentence?

    a. School
    b. Store
    c. He
    d. After

English and Language Usage

6. He was exhausted and very tired when he finally finished the exam.

What part of this sentence is redundant?

    a. finished the exam
    b. He was exhausted
    c. And very tired
    d. When he finally

7. Choose the sentence with the correct usage.

    a. The ceremony had an emotional effect on the groom, but the bride was not affected.
    b. The ceremony had an emotional affect on the groom, but the bride was not affected.
    c. The ceremony had an emotional effect on the groom, but the bride was not effected.
    d. The ceremony had an emotional affect on the groom, but the bride was not affected.

8. I never want to speak to him again!

What type of sentence is this?

    a. Imperative
    b. Interrogative
    c. Exclamatory
    d. Declarative

9. Choose the correct sentence.

    a. Each boy and girl were given a toy.
    b. Each boy and girl was given a toy.
    c. Each boy and girl is given a toy.
    d. None of the above.

10. He went to the store after school.

What is the simple predicate of the sentence?

    a. Went to the store
    b. After school
    c. He
    d. He went

11. Choose the sentence with the correct usage.

a. Anna was taller then Luis, but then he grew four inches in three months.
b. Anna was taller then Luis, but than he grew four inches in three months.
c. Anna was taller than Luis, but than he grew four inches in three months.
d. Anna was taller than Luis, but then he grew four inches in three months.

12. Sarah bought some <u>stationeries</u>.

Choose the correct word to replace the underlined word above.

a. stationary
b. stationarys
c. stationaryes
d. none of the above

13. I have two <u>son-in-laws</u>.

Choose the correct word to replace the underlined word above.

a. sons-in-laws
b. sons-on-law
c. sons-in-law
d. none of the above

14. Choose the sentence with the correct grammar.

a. Mathematics were my best subject in school
b. Mathematics are my best subject in school
c. Mathematics was my best subject in school
d. None of the above

Fill in the Blank.

15. All the people at the school, including the teachers and _____ were glad when summer break came.

a. students:
b. students,
c. students;
d. students

English and Language Usage

16. My wife's brother is a good friend and my brother-in-law.

What part of this sentence is redundant?

    a. Is a good friend

    b. And my brother-in-law

    c. Good friend and my brother-in-law

    d. There is no redundancy in this sentence

17. Choose the sentence with the correct grammar.

    a. The tongs are now hot enough

    b. The tongs is now hot enough

    c. Both of the above

    d. None of the above

18. The Ford Motor Company was named for Henry Ford, _____.

    a. which had founded the company.

    b. who founded the company.

    c. whose had founded the company.

    d. whom had founded the company.

19. Choose the sentence with the correct grammar.

    a. He would have postponed the camping trip, if he would have known about the forecast.

    b. If he would have known about the forecast, he would have postponed the camping trip.

    c. If he have known about the forecast, he would have postponed the camping trip.

    d. If he had known about the forecast, he would have postponed the camping trip.

20. Choose the correct sentence.

    a. Shakespeare wrote more than 37 Plays, including Much Ado about Nothing.

    b. Shakespeare wrote more than 37 plays, including Much ado about nothing.

    c. Shakespeare wrote more than 37 plays, including Much Ado about Nothing.

    d. Shakespeare wrote more than 37 Plays, including Much Ado About Nothing.

21. Choose the correct spelling.

   a. arguemint
   b. arguement
   c. argument
   d. arguemant

22. Choose the correct spelling.

   a. occurrence
   b. ocurrence
   c. occurence
   d. ocurence

23. Choose the correct spelling.

   a. desparate
   b. desperete
   c. desperate
   d. despirate

24. Sit up straight ____

   a. ;
   b. ?
   c. .
   d. :

25. They asked what time the department store would open ____

   a. ?
   b. .
   c. ,
   d. ;

English and Language Usage

26. Who do you think will win the contest _____

    a. .
    b. !
    c. ?
    d. ,

27. The <u>lazy</u> brown fox jumper over the sleeping dog.

What part of speech is the underlined word?

    a. Noun
    b. Verb
    c. Adjective
    d. Adverb

28. The <u>tall</u> buildings blocked out the sun.

What part of speech is the underlined word?

    a. Noun
    b. Verb
    c. Adjective
    d. Adverb

29. Which of the following sentences contains a redundant phrase?

    a. I filled the tank to capacity.
    b. At the moment, she is getting ready.
    c. I won't be there for several minutes
    d. None of the above

30. Choose the correct sentence.

    a. They said it is going to rain on the radio.
    b. They said on the radio it is going to rain.
    c. They are going to say it is going to rain on the radio.
    d. None of the above.

Answer Key

1. A
Felony: A serious criminal offense, which, under federal law, is punishable by death or imprisonment for a term exceeding one year.

2. A
The cardinal directions, North, South East and West are capitalized. In general, the first letter is capitalized for well-defined regions, e.g. South America, Lower California, Tennessee Valley. This general rule also applies to zones of the Earth's surface (North Temperate Zone, the Equator). In other cases, do not capitalize the points of the compass (north China, south-east London) or other adjectives (western Arizona, central New Mexico, upper Yangtze, lower Rio Grande)

3. B
Palatial: Of or relating to a palace.

4. C
Underlings: A subordinate, or person of lesser rank or authority.

5. C
'He' is the subject of the sentence.

6. C
The phrase, 'and very tired' is redundant after saying he was exhausted.

7. A
"Affect" is a verb, while "effect" is a noun.

8. C
This is an exclamatory sentence.

9. B
Use the singular verb form when nouns are qualified with "every" or "each," even if they are joined by 'and.'

10. A
The simple predicate is the action being performed by the subject.

11. D
"Than" is used for comparison. "Then" is used to indicate a point in time.

12. A
"Stationary" is both the singular and plural forms.

13. C
The correct form is son-in-law in the singular and sons-in-law in the plural.

English and Language Usage

14. C
Always use the singular verb form for nouns like politics, wages, mathematics, innings, news, advice, summons, furniture, information, poetry, machinery, vacation, scenery etc.

15. B
The comma separates a phrase.

16. B
'And my brother-in-law' is redundant since we already know he is his wife's brother.

17. A
Use a plural verb for nouns like measles, tongs, trousers, riches, scissors etc.

18. B
The sentence refers to a person, so "who" is the only correct option.

19. D
The third conditional is used for talking about an unreal situation (a situation that did not happen) in the past. For example, "If I had studied harder, [if clause] I would have passed the exam [main clause]. This has the same meaning as, "I failed the exam because I didn't study hard enough."

20. C
The names of plays are capitalized. All words except articles are capitalized.

21. C
Argument is the correct spelling.

22. A
Occurrence is the correct spelling.

23. C
Desperate is the correct spelling.

24. C
A period or an exclamation mark are to end an imperative sentence, that is, at the end of a direction or a command.

25. B
A period is used to end an indirect question. An indirect question is always a part of a declarative sentence and it does not require an answer.

26. C
A question mark is used to end an interrogative sentence, that is, at the end of a direct question which requires an answer.

27. D
The underlined word, lazy, is an adverb. Adverbs are words or phrases that modify or

qualify an adjective, verb, or other adverb or a phrase.

28. C
'Tall' in this sentence is an adjective. Adjectives are words or phrases naming an attribute, added to, or grammatically related to a noun to modify or describe it.

29. A
If the tank is filled, it is filled to capacity, so describing something as "filled to capacity" is redundant.

30. B
The correct sentence is, "They said on the radio it is going to rain." The first choice, "They said it is going to rain on the radio," means it is going to rain on the radio.

English Grammar and Punctuation Tutorials

Capitalization

Although many of the rules for capitalization are pretty straight forward, there are several tricky points that are important to review.

Starting a Sentence

Everyone knows that you need to capitalize the first letter of the first word in a sentence, but is it really all that easy to figure out where one sentence starts and another stops? Take these three examples:

That was the moment it really sunk in: There would be no hockey this year.

It was April and that could mean only one thing: baseball.

We played for hours before heading home; everyone felt tired and happy.

In the first example, the first letter after the colon is capitalized while in the second example, it is not. That is because everything after the first example's colon is a complete sentence, while, after the second example, there is only one word. In example three you have what could be a complete sentence ("everyone felt tired and happy"), but which is not because it follows a semicolon, making it just another clause instead.

Within a sentence you can have an additional complete sentence if the sentence follows a colon. However, if what could be a complete sentence follows a semicolon, it is a clause and does not get capitalized.

Remember that the same rules apply for quotation marks that apply for colons: A complete sentence inside quotation marks is capitalized, but a single word or phrase is not.

Proper Nouns

The first letter of all proper nouns needs to be capitalized. There are many categories of proper noun. The most common proper nouns are the specific names of people (such as Bill), places (such as Germany) or things (such as Honda Civic). However, there are several less obvious categories of words that should be capitalized as proper nouns.

Historical events such as World War II or the California Gold Rush need to be capitalized.

The names of celestial bodies such as Orion's Belt need to be capitalized.

The names of ethnicities such as African American or Hispanic need to be capitalized.

Relationship words that replace a person's name such as Mom, Doctor and Mister need to be capitalized. However, this only happens when you use the word to replace the person's name. In the sentence, "My mom went to the store," you do not capitalize it, while in the sentence, "Hey Mom, did you get toothpaste at the store?" you do capitalize it.

Geographical locations are capitalized. This can get tricky because capitalized geographical locations and non-capitalized directions are easy to confuse. Saying, "We drove south for hours," is a direction, so the word "south" should not be capitalized. However, when saying, "While in the United States, we drove to the South to look at Civil War battle fields," you do capitalize the word "South." The difference is that in the first sentence "south" is just the direction you drove. In the second sentence "the South" is a specific region of the United States that formed itself into the Confederacy during the US Civil War.

Proper Adjectives

Proper adjectives are the adjective forms of proper nouns. People from Germany are German; people from Canada are Canadian. German and Canadian are proper adjectives because they are forms of proper nouns that are used to describe other nouns.

Titles of Works

Titles of works are generally capitalized following a specific pattern. Capitalize all the important words in a sentence. Do not capitalize unimportant words such as prepositions and articles.

For example: Alien Spaceship Spotted over Many of the World's Capitals

Notice that the prepositions "over" and "of," and the article "the" are the only non-capitalized words in the sentence.

Colons and Semicolons

Within a sentence there are several different types of punctuation marks that can denote a pause. Each of these punctuation marks has different rules when it comes to its structure and usage, so we will look at each one in turn.

Colons

The colon is used primarily to introduce information. A colon can start lists such as in the sentence, "There were several things Susan had to get at the store: bread, cereal, lettuce and tomatoes." Or a colon be used to point out specific information, such as in the sentence, "It was only then that the group fully realized what had happened: The Martian invasion had begun."

Note that if the information after the colon is a complete sentence, you capitalize and punctuate it exactly like you would a sentence. If, however, it does not constitute a complete sentence, you don't have to capitalize anything. ("Peering out the window Meredith saw them: zombies.")

Semicolons

Semicolon can be thought of as super commas. They denote a stronger stop than a comma does, but they are still weaker than a period, not quite capable of ending a sentence. Semicolons are primarily used to separate independent clauses that are not being separated by a coordinating conjunction. ("Chris went to the store; he bought chips and salsa.") Semicolons can only do this, however, when the ideas in each clause are related. For instance, the sentence, "It's raining outside; my sister went to the movies," is not a proper usage of the semicolon since those clauses have nothing to do with each other.

Semicolons can also be used in lists if one or more element in the list is itself made up of a smaller list. If you want to write a list of things you plan to bring to a picnic, and those things only include a Frisbee, a chair and some pasta salad, you would not need to use a semicolon. However, if you also wanted to bring plastic knives, forks and spoons, you would need to write your sentence like this: "For our picnic I am bringing a Frisbee; a chair; plastic knives, forks and spoons; and some pasta salad."

This example of semicolon use preserves the smaller list that you have in your larger list.

Comma

Commas are probably the most commonly used punctuation mark in English. Commas can break the flow of writing to give it a more natural sounding style, and they are the main punctuation mark used to separate ideas. Commas also separate lists, introductory adverbs, introductory prepositional phrases, dates and addresses.

English and Language Usage

The most rigid way that comma are used is when separating clauses. There are two primary types of clauses in a sentence, independent and subordinate (sometimes called dependent). Independent clauses are clauses that express a complete thought, such as, "Tim went to the store." Subordinate clauses, on the other hand, only express partial thoughts which expand on an independent clause, such as, "after the game ended," which you can see is clearly not a complete sentence. (You will learn more about clauses in different lessons.)

The rule for commas with clauses is that a comma must separate the clauses when a subordinate clause comes first in a sentence: "After the game ended, Tim went to the store." But there should not be a comma when a subordinate clause follows an independent clause: "Tim went to the store after the game ended." If you leave the comma out of the first example, you have a run-on sentence. If you add one into the second example, you have a comma-splice error. Also, when you have two independent clauses joined with a coordinating conjunction, you need to separate them with a comma. "Tim went to the store, and Beth went home."

There are some artistic exceptions to these rules, such as adding a pause for literary effect, but for the most part, they are set in stone.

Commas are also used to separate items in a list. This area of English is unfortunately less clear than it should be, with two separate rules depending on what standard you are following. To understand the two different rules, let's pretend you are having a party at your house, and you are making a list of refreshments your friends will want. You may decide to serve three things: 1) pizza 2) chips 3) drinks. There are two different rules governing how you should punctuate this. According to many grammar books, you would write this as, "At the store I will buy pizza, chips, and drinks." This variation puts a comma after each item in the list. It is the version that the style books used in most college English and history courses will prefer, so it is probably the one you should follow. However, the Associated Press style guide, which is used in college journalism classes and at newspapers and magazines, says the sentence should be written like this: "At the store I will buy pizza, chips and drinks." Here you only use a comma between the first two words, letting the word "and" act as the separator between the last two.

Another important place to use commas is when you have a modifier that describes an element of a sentence, but that does not directly follow the thing it describes. Look at the sentence: "Tim went over to visit Beth, watching the full moon along the way." In this sentence there is no confusion about who is "watching the full moon"; it is Tim, probably as he walks to Beth's house. If you remove the comma, however, you get this: "Tim went over to visit Beth watching the full moon along the way." Now it sounds as though Beth is watching the full moon, and we are forced to wonder what "way" the moon is traveling along.

Commas are also used when adding introductory prepositional phrases and introductory adverbs to sentences. A comma is always needed following an introductory adverb. ("Quickly, Jody ran to the car.") Commas are even necessary when you have an adverb introducing a clause within a sentence, even if the clause not the first clause of the sentence. ("Amanda wanted to go to the movie; however, she knew her homework was more important.")

With introductory prepositional phrases you only add a comma if the phrase (or if a group of introductory phrases) is five or more words long. Thus, the sentence you just read did not have a comma following its introductory prepositional phrase ("With introductory prepositional phrases") because it was only four words. Compare that to this sentence with a five word introductory phrase: "After the ridiculously long class, the friends needed to relax."

The last main way that comma are used in sentences is to separate out information that does not need to be there. For instance, "My cousin Hector, who wore a blue hat at the party, thought you were funny." The fact that Hector wore a blue hat is interesting, but it is not vital to the sentence; it could be removed and not changed the sentence's meaning. Therefore, it gets commas around it. Along these lines you should remember that any clause introduced by the word that is considered to provide essential information to the sentence and should not get commas around it. Conversely, any clause starting with the word which is considered nonessential and should not get commas around it.

How to Answer English Grammar Multiple Choice - Verb Tense

This tutorial is designed to help you answer English Grammar multiple choice questions as well as a very quick refresher on verb tenses. It is assumed that you have some familiarity with the verb tenses covered here. If you find these questions difficulty or do not understand the tense construction, we recommend you seek out additional instruction.

Tenses Covered

1. Past Progressive
2. Present Perfect
3. Present Perfect Progressive
4. Present Progressive
5. Simple Future
6. Simple Future – "Going to" Form
7. Past Perfect Progressive
8. Future Perfect Progressive
9. Future Perfect
10. Future Progressive
11. Past Perfect

English and Language Usage

1. The Past Progressive Tense

How to Recognize This Tense

He *was running* very fast when he fell.

They *were drinking* coffee when he arrived.

About the Past Progressive Tense

This tense is used to speak of an action that was in progress in the past when another event occurred.

The action was unfolding at a point in the past.

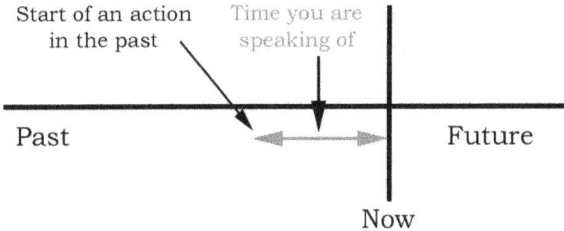

Past Progressive Tense Construction

This tense is formed by using the past tense of the verb "to be" plus the present participle of the main verb.

Sample Question

Bill _____ lunch when we arrived.

    a. will eat
    b. is eating
    c. eats
    d. was eating

How to Answer This Type of Question

1. First examine the question for clues about the time frame.

The sentence ends with "when we arrived," so we know the time frame is a point ("when") in the past (arrived).

The correct answer will refer to an ongoing action at a point of time in the past.

2. Examine the choices and eliminate any obviously incorrect answers.

Choice A is the future tense so we can eliminate.

Choice B is the present continuous so we can eliminate.

Choice C is present tense so we can eliminate.

Choice D refers to an action that takes place at a point of time in the past ("was eating").

2. The Present Perfect Tense

How to Recognize This Tense

I *have had* enough to eat.

We *have been* to Paris many times.

I *have known* him for five years.

I *have been* coming here since I was a child.

About the Present Perfect Tense

This tense expresses the idea that something happened (or didn't happen) at an unspecific time in the past, until the present. The action happened at an unspecified time in the past. (If there is a specific time mentioned, the simple past tense is used.) It can be used for repeated action, accomplishments, changes over time and uncompleted action.

English and Language Usage

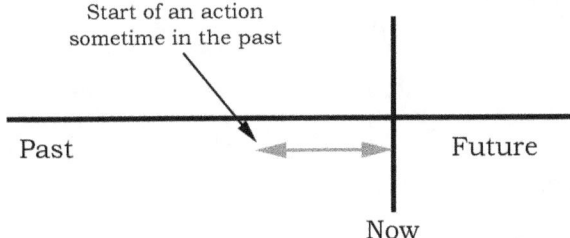

Present Perfect Tense Construction

It is also used with "for" and "since."

This tense is formed by using the present tense of the verb "to have" plus the past participle of the main verb.

Sample Question

I _____ these birds many times.

    a. am seeing

    b. will saw

    c. have seen

    d. have saw

How to Answer This Type of Question

1. First examine the question for clues about the time frame.

"Many times" tells us that the action is repeated and in the past.

2. Examine the choices and eliminate any obviously incorrect answers.

Choice A, "am seeing" is incorrect because it is a continuing action, i.e. in the present; it also doesn't use a form of 'have'.

Choice B is grammatically incorrect.

Choice C tells of something that has happened in the past and is now over. Best choice so far.

Choice D is grammatically incorrect.

3. The Present Perfect Progressive Tense

How to Recognize This Tense

We *have been seeing* a lot of rainy days.

I *have been reading* some very good books.

About the Present Perfect Progressive Tense

This tense expresses the idea that something happened (or didn't happen) in the relatively recent past, but <u>the action is not finished.</u> It is used to express the duration of the action.

NOTE: The present perfect speaks of an action that happened sometime in the past, but this action is finished. In the present perfect progressive tense, the action that started in the past is still going on.

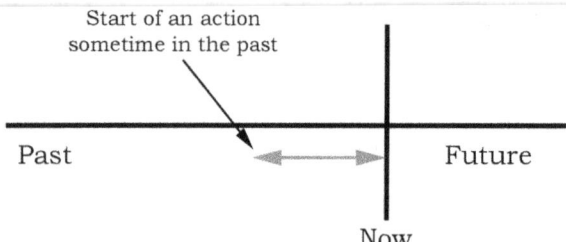

Present Perfect Progressive Tense Construction

This tense is formed by using the present tense of the verb "to have," plus "been," plus the present participle of the main verb.

Sample Question

Bill _____ there for two hours.

    a. sits

    b. sitting

    c. has been sitting

    d. will sat

How to Answer This Type of Question

1. First examine the question for clues about the time frame.

"For two hours" tells us that the action, "sits," is continuous up to now, and may continue into the future.

English and Language Usage

Note this sentence could also be the simple past tense,

Bill sat there for two hours.

Or the future tense,

Bill will sit there for two hours.

However, these are not among the options.

2. Examine the choices and eliminate any obviously incorrect answers.

Choice A is incorrect because it is the present tense.
Choice B is incorrect because it is the present continuous. Choice C is correct. "Has been sitting" expresses a continuous action in the past that isn't finished.
Choice D is grammatically incorrect.

4. The Present Progressive Tense

How to Recognize This Tense

We *are having* a delicious lunch.

They *are driving* much too fast.

About the Present Progressive Tense

This tense is used to express what the action is <u>right now</u>. The action started in the recent past, and is continuing into the future.

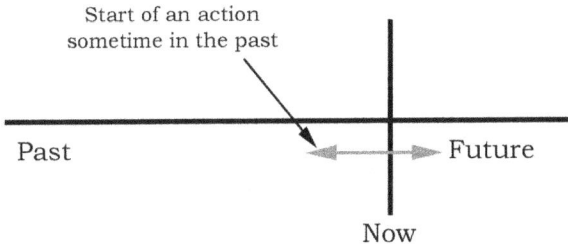

Present Perfect Tense Construction

The Present Progressive Tense is formed by using the present tense of "to be" plus the present participle of the main verb.

Sample Question

She _____ very hard these days.

    a. works

    b. is working

    c. will work

    d. worked

How to Answer This Type of Question

1. First examine the question for clues about the time frame.

The end of the sentence includes "these days" which tell us the action started in the past, continues into the present, and may continue into the future.

2. Examine the choices and eliminate any obviously incorrect answers.

Choice A, the simple present is incorrect.
Choice B, "is working" is correct.
Check the other two choices just to be sure. Choice C is future tense, and choice D is past tense, so they can be eliminated.

The correct answer is choice B.

5. The Simple Future Tense

How to Recognize This Tense

I *will see* you tomorrow.
We *will drive* the car.

About the Simple Future Tense

This tense shows that the action will happen some time in the future.

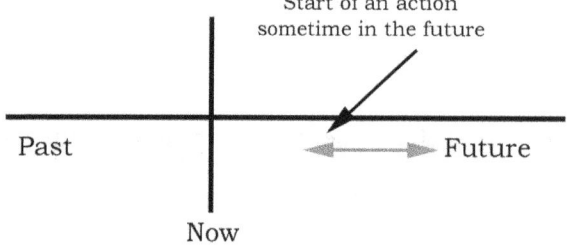

ENGLISH AND LANGUAGE USAGE

Simple Future Tense Construction

The tense is formed by using "will" plus the root form of the verb. (The root form of the verb is the infinitive without "to." Examples: read, swim.)

Sample Question

We _____ to Paris next year.

    a. went

    b. had been

    c. will go

    d. go

How to Answer This Type of Question

1. First examine the question for clues about the time frame.

The last two words of the sentence, "next year," clearly identify this sentence as referring to the future.

2. Examine the choices and eliminate any obviously incorrect answers.

Choice A is the past tense and can be eliminated.

Choice B is the past perfect tense and can be eliminated.

Choice D is the simple present and can be eliminated.

Choice C is the only one left and is the correct simple future tense.

6. The Simple Future Tense – The "Going to" Form

How to Recognize This Tense

I *am going to* see you tomorrow.

We *are going to* drive the car.

About the Simple Future Tense

This form of the future tense is used to show the intention of doing something in the future. (This is the strict grammatical meaning, but in daily speech, it is often used interchangeably with the simple future tense, the "will" form.)

The tense is formed by using the present conditional tense of "to go," plus the infinitive of the verb.

Sample Question

I _____ shopping in an hour.

    a. go
    b. have gone
    c. am going to go
    d. went

How to Answer This Type of Question

1. First examine the question for clues about the time frame.

"In an hour" clearly identifies the action as taking place in the future.

2. Examine the choices and eliminate any obviously incorrect answers.

Choice A is the simple present tense and be eliminated.

Choice B is the past perfect and can be eliminated.

Choice C is the correct answer.

Choice D is the past tense and can be eliminated.

7. The Past Perfect Progressive Tense

How to Recognize This Tense

I *had been sleeping* for an hour when you phoned.

We *had been eating* our dinner when they all came into the dining room.

About the Past Perfect Progressive Tense

This tense is used to show that the action had been going on for a period of time in the past when another action, also in the past, occurred.

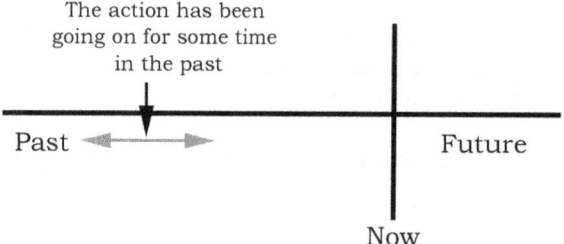

Past Perfect Tense Construction

The tense is formed by using the past perfect tense of the verb "to be" plus the present participle of the main verb.

Sample Question

How long _____ you _____ when I saw you?

    a. are ____ running

    b. had ____ running

    c. had ____ been running

    d. was ____ running

How to Answer This Type of Question

1. First examine the question for clues about the time frame.

"When I saw" tells us the sentence happened at a point of time ("when") in the past ("saw").

2. Examine the choices and eliminate any obviously incorrect answers.

Choice A, "are running" is incorrect and can be eliminated.

Choice B, "Had ___ running" is grammatically incorrect and can be eliminated.

Choice C is correct.

Choice D is grammatically incorrect so the answer is Choice C.

8. Future Perfect Progressive Tense

How to Recognize This Tense

I *will have been working* here for two years in March.

I *will have been driving* for four hours when I get there, so I will be tired.

About the Future Perfect Progressive Tense

This tense is used to show that the action continues up to a point of time in the future.

Future Prefect Progressive Tense Construction

This tense is formed by using the future perfect tense of "to be" plus the present participle of the main verb.

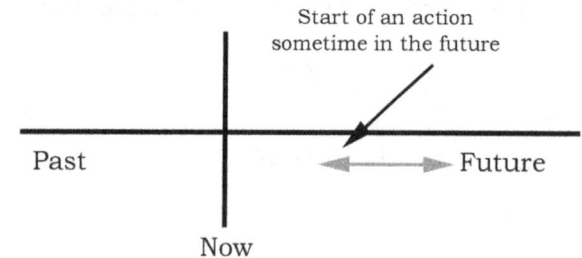

Sample Question

_____ you _____ all the time I am gone?

    a. have _____ been working

    b. will _____ have been working

    c. are _____ worked

    d. will _____ worked

How to Answer This Type of Question

1. First examine the question for clues about the time frame.

"All the time I am gone" refers to an action in the future ("time I am gone") and the action is progressive ("all the time"). The progressive action means the correct choice will be a verb tense that ends in "ing."

2. Examine the choices and eliminate any obviously incorrect answers.

Choice A, the past perfect, refers to a past continuous event and is also grammatically incorrect in the sentence, so Choice A can be eliminated.

Choice B looks correct because it refers to an action will be going on for a period of time in the future.

Examine Choices C and D just to be sure. Both choices are grammatically incorrect and can be eliminated.
Choice B is the correct answer.

English and Language Usage

9. The Future Perfect Tense

How to Recognize This Tense

By next November, I *will have received* my promotion.

By the time he gets home, she is going *to have cleaned* the entire house.

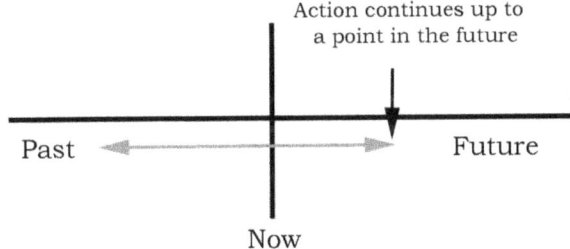

About the Future Perfect Tense

The future perfect tense expresses action in the future before another action in the future. This is the past in the future. For example:

He *will have prepared* dinner when she arrives.

Future Perfect Tense Construction

This tense is formed by "will + have + past participle."

Sample Question

They _____ their seats before the game begins.

    a. will have find
    b. will find
    c. will have found
    d. found

How to Answer This Type of Question

1. First examine the question for clues about the time frame.

This question could be several different tenses. The only clue about the time frame is "before the game begins," which refers to a specific point of time.

We know it isn't in the past, because "begins" is incorrect for the past tense. Similarly with the present. So the question is about something that happens in the future, before another event in the future.

2. Examine the choices and eliminate any obviously incorrect answers.

Choice A can be eliminated as incorrect.
Choice B looks good, so mark it and check the others before making a final decision.
Choice C is the past perfect and can be eliminated because the time frame is incorrect.
Choice D is the simple past tense and can be eliminated for the same reason.

10. Future Progressive Tense

How to Recognize This Tense

The teams *will be playing* soccer when we arrive.

At 3:45 the soccer fans *will be waiting* for the game to start at 4:00 o'clock

At 3:45 the soccer players *will be preparing* to play at 4:00 o'clock

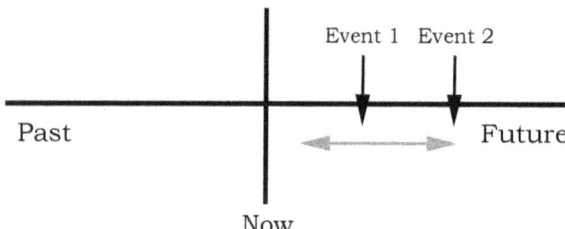

About the Future Progressive Tense

The future progressive tense talks about a continuing action in the future.

Future Progressive Tense Construction

will + be + (root form) + ing = will be playing

Sample Question

Many excited fans _____ a bus to see the game at 4:00.

    a. catch
    b. catching
    c. have been catching
    d. will be catching

English and Language Usage

How to Answer This Type of Question

1. First examine the question for clues about the time frame.

"At 4:00," tells us the sentence is either in the past OR in the future.

2. Examine the choices and eliminate any obviously incorrect answers.

From the time frame of the sentence, the answer will be past or future tense.

Choice A is the present tense and can be eliminated.
Choice B is the present continuous tense and can be eliminated.
Choice C is the past perfect continuous and can be eliminated.
Choice D is the only one left. Quickly examining the tense, it is future progressive and is correct in the sentence.

11. The Past Perfect Tense

How to Recognize This Tense

The party *had* just *started* when the coach arrived.

We *had waited* for twenty minutes when the bus finally came.

About the Past Perfect

The past perfect tense talks about two events that happened in the past and establishes which event happened first.

Another example is, "We had eaten when he arrived."

The two events are "eat" and "he arrived." From the sentence above the past perfect tense tells us the first event, "eat" happened before the second event, "he arrived."

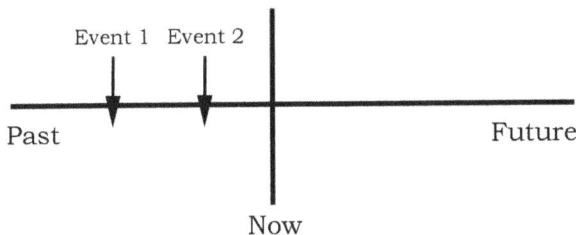

I had already eaten when my friends arrived.

Past Perfect Tense Construction

The past perfect is formed by "have" plus the past participle.

Sample Question

It was time to go home after they _____ the game.

    a. will win
    b. win
    c. had won
    d. wins

How to Answer This Type of Question

1. First examine the question for clues about the time frame.

"Was" tells us the sentence happened in the past. Also notice there are two events, "go home" and "after the game."

2. Examine the choices and eliminate any obviously incorrect answers.

Choice A is the future tense and can be eliminated. Choice B is the simple present and can be eliminated. Choice C is the past perfect and orders the two events in the past. Choice D is the present tense and incorrect and can be eliminated, so choice C is the correct answer.

Common English Usage Mistakes - A Quick Review

Like some parts of English grammar, usage is definitely going to be on the exam and there isn't any tricky strategies or shortcuts to help you get through this section. Here is a quick review of common usage mistakes.

1. May and Might

'May' can act as a principal verb, which can express permission or possibility.

Examples:

Lets wait, the meeting may have started.
May I begin now?

'May' can act as an auxiliary verb, which expresses a purpose or wish

Examples:

May you find favour in the sight of your employer.

May your wishes come true.
People go to school so that they may be educated.

The past tense of may is might.

Examples:

I asked if I might begin

'Might' signifies a weak or slim possibility or polite suggestion.

Examples:

You might find him in his office, but I doubt it.
You might offer to help if you want to.

2. Lie and Lay

The verb lay should always take an object. The three forms of the verb lay are: laid, lay and laid.

The verb lie (recline) should not take any object. The three forms of the verb lie are: lay, lie and lain.

Examples:

Lay on the bed.
The tables were laid by the students.
Let the little kid lie.
The patient lay on the table.

The dog has lain there for 30 minutes.

Note: The verb lie can also mean "to tell a falsehood." This verb can appear in three forms: lied, lie, and lied. This is different from the verb lie (recline) mentioned above.

Examples:

The accused is fond of telling lies.
Did she lie?

3. Would and should

The past tense of shall is 'should', and so "should" generally follows the same principles as "shall."

The past tense of will is "would," and so "would" generally follows the same principles as "will."

The two verbs 'would and should' can be correctly used interchangeably to signify obligation. The two verbs also have some unique uses too. Should is used in three persons to signify obligation.

Examples:

I should go after work.
People should do exercises everyday.
You should be generous.

"Would" is specially used in any of the three persons, to signify willingness, determination and habitual action.

Examples:

They would go for a test run every Saturday.
They would not ignore their duties.
She would try to be punctual.

4. Principle and Auxiliary Verbs

Two principle verbs can be used along with one auxiliary verb as long as the auxiliary verb form suits the two principal verbs.

Examples:

A number of people have been employed and some promoted.

A new tree has been planted and the old has been cut down.

Again note the difference in the verb form.

5. Can and Could

A. Can is used to express capacity or ability.

English and Language Usage

Examples:

I can complete the assignment today
He can meet up with his target.

B. Can is also used to express permission.

Examples:

Yes, you can begin

In the sentence below, "can" was used to mean the same thing as "may." However, the difference is that the word "can" is used for negative or interrogative sentences, while "may" is used in affirmative sentences to express possibility.

Examples:

They may be correct.   Positive sentence - use may.
Can this statement be correct? A question using "can."
It cannot be correct. Negative sentence using "can."

The past tense of can is could. It can serve as a principal verb when it is used to express its own meaning.

Examples:

Despite the difficulty of the test, he could still perform well.
"Could" here is used to express ability.

6. Ought

The verb ought should normally be followed by the word to.

Examples:

I *ought to* close shop now.

The verb 'ought' can be used to express:

A. Desirability

You ought to wash your hands before eating.   It is desirable to wash your hands.

B. Probability

She ought to be on her way back by now.   She is probably on her way.

C. Moral obligation or duty

The government ought to protect the oppressed.   It is the government's duty to protect the oppressed.

7. Raise and Rise

Rise
The verb rise means to go up, or to ascend.
The verb rise can appear in three forms, rose, rise, and risen. The verb should not take an object.

Examples:

The bird rose very slowly.
The trees rise above the house.
My aunt has risen in her career.

Raise
The verb raise means to increase, to lift up.
The verb raise can appear in three forms, raised, raise and raised.

Examples:

He raised his hand.
The workers requested a raise.
Do not raise that subject.

8. Past Tense and Past Participle

Pay attention to the proper use these verbs: sing, show, ring, awake, fly, flow, begin, hang and sink.

Mistakes usually occur when using the past participle and past tense of these verbs as they are often mixed up.

Each of these verbs can appear in three forms:

Sing, Sang, Sung.
Show, Showed, Showed/Shown.
Ring, Rang, Rung.
Awake, awoke, awaken

Fly, Flew, Flown.
Flow, Flowed, Flowed.
Begin, Began, Begun.
Hang, Hanged, Hanged (a criminal)
Hang, Hung, Hung (a picture)
Sink, Sank, Sunk.

Examples:

The stranger rang the door bell. (simple past tense)
I have rung the door bell already. (past participle - an action completed in the past)

The stone sank in the river. (simple past tense)
The stone had already sunk. (past participle - an action completed in the past)

The meeting began at 4:00.
The meeting has begun.

9. Shall and Will

When speaking informally, the two can be used interchangeably. In formal writing, they must be used correctly.

"Will" is used in the second or third person, while "shall" is used in the first person. Both verbs are used to express a time or even in the future.

Examples:

I shall, We shall (First Person)
You will (Second Person)
They will (Third Person)

This principle however reverses when the verbs are to be used to express threats, determination, command, willingness, promise or compulsion. In these instances, will is now used in first person and shall in the second and third person.

Examples:

I will be there next week, no matter what.
This is a promise, so the first person "I" takes "will."

You shall ensure that the work is completed.
This is a command, so the second person "you" takes "shall."

I will try to make payments as promised.
This is a promise, so the first person "I" takes "will."

They shall have arrived by the end of the day.

This is a determination, so the third person "they" takes shall.

Note
A. The two verbs, shall and will should not occur twice in the same sentence when the same future is being referred to

Example:

I shall arrive early if my driver is here on time.

B. Will should not be used in the first person when questions are being asked

Examples:

Shall I go ?
Shall we go?

Subject Verb Agreement

Verbs in any sentence must agree with the subject of the sentence both in person and number. Problems usually occur when the verb doesn't correspond with the right subject or the verb fails to match the noun close to it.

Unfortunately, there is no easy way around these principles - no tricky strategy or easy rule. You just have to memorize them.

Here is a quick review:

The verb to be, present (past)

Person	Singular	Plural
First	I am (was)	we are (were)
Second	you are (were)	you are (were)
Third	he, she, it is (was)	they are (were)

The verb to have, present (past)

English and Language Usage

Person	Singular	Plural
First	I have (had)	we have (had)
Second	you have (had)	you have (had)
Third	he, she, it has (had)	they have (had)

Regular verbs, e.g. to walk, present (past)

Person	Singular	Plural
First	I walk (walked)	we walk (walked)
Second	you walk (walked)	you walk (walked)
Third	he, she, it walks (walked)	they work (walked)

1. Every and Each

When nouns are qualified by "every" or "each," they take a singular verb even if they are joined by 'and'

Examples:

Each mother and daughter *was* a given separate test.
Every teacher and student *was* properly welcomed.

2. Plural Nouns

Nouns like measles, tongs, trousers, riches, scissors etc. are all plural.

Examples:

The trousers *are* dirty.
My scissors *have* gone missing.
The tongs *are* on the table.

3. With and As Well

Two subjects linked by "with" or "as well" should have a verb that matches the first subject.

Examples:

The pencil, with the papers and equipment, *is* on the desk.
David as well as Louis is coming.

4. Plural Nouns

The following nouns take a singular verb:

>politics, mathematics, innings, news, advice, summons, furniture, information, poetry, machinery, vacation, scenery

Examples:

The machinery *is* difficult to assemble
The furniture *has* been delivered
The scenery *was* beautiful

5. Single Entities

A proper noun in plural form that refers to a single entity requires a singular verb. This is a complicated way of saying; some things appear to be plural, but are really singular, or some nouns refer to a collection of things but the collection is really singular.

Examples:

The United Nations Organization *is* the decision maker in the matter.

Here the "United Nations Organization" is really only one "thing" or noun, but is made up of many "nations."

The book, "The Seven Virgins" *was* not available in the library.

Here there is only one book, although the title of the book is plural.

6. Specific Amounts are always singular

A plural noun that refers to a specific amount or quantity that is considered as a whole (dozen, hundred, score etc) requires a singular verb.

Examples:

60 minutes *is* quite a long time.
Here "60 minutes" is considered a whole, and therefore one item (singular noun).

The first million is the most difficult.

7. Either, Neither and Each are always singular

The verb is always singular when used with: either, each, neither, every one and many.

Examples:

Either of the boys *is* lying.
Each of the employees *has* been well compensated
Many a police officer *has* been found to be courageous
Every one of the teachers *is* responsible

8. Linking with Either, Or, and Neither match the second subject

Two subjects linked by "either," "or," "nor" or "neither" should have a verb that matches the second subject.

Examples:

Neither David nor Paul *will* be coming.
Either Mary or Tina *is* paying.

Note
If one subject linked by "either," "or," "nor" or "neither" is in plural form, then the verb should also be in plural, and the verb should be close to the plural subject.

Examples:
Neither the mother *nor* her kids *have* eaten.
Either Mary *or* her *friends are* paying.

9. Collective Nouns are Plural

Some collective nouns such as poultry, gentry, cattle, vermin etc. are considered plural and require a plural verb.

Examples:

The *poultry are* sick.
The *cattle are* well fed.

Note
Collective nouns involving people can work with both plural and singular verbs.

Examples:

Nigerians are known to be hard working
Europeans live in Africa

10. Nouns that are Singular and Plural

Nouns like deer, sheep, swine, salmon etc. can be singular or plural and require the same verb form.

Examples:

The swine is feeding. (singular)
The swine are feeding. (plural)

The salmon is on the table. (singular)
The salmon are running upstream. (plural)

11. Collective Nouns are Singular

Collective nouns such as Army, Jury, Assembly, Committee, Team etc should carry a singular verb when they subscribe to one idea. If the ideas or views are more than one, then the verb used should be plural.

Examples:

The committee is in agreement in their decision.

The committee were in disagreement in their decision.
The jury has agreed on a verdict.
The jury were unable to agree on a verdict.

English and Language Usage

12. Subjects links by "and" are plural.

Two subjects linked by "and" always require a plural verb

Examples:

David and John are students.

Note
If the subjects linked by "and" are used as one phrase, or constitute one idea, then the verb must be singular

The color of his socks and shoe is black.
Here "socks and shoe" are two nouns, however the subject is "color" which is singular.

Help with Building your Vocabulary

Vocabulary tests can be daunting when you think of the enormous number of words that might come up in the exam. As the exam date draws near, your anxiety will grow because you know that, no matter how many words you memorize, chances are, you will still remember so few. Here are some tips which you can use to hurdle the big words that may come up in your exam without having to open the dictionary and memorize all the words known to humankind.

Build up and tear apart the big words. Big words, like many other things, are composed of small parts. Some words are made up of many other words. A man who lifts weights for example, is a weight lifter. Words are also made up of word parts called prefixes, suffixes and roots. Often times, we can see the relationship of different words through these parts. A person who is skilled with both hands is ambidextrous. A word with double meaning is ambiguous. A person with two conflicting emotions is ambivalent. Two words with synonymous meanings often have the same root. Bio, a root word derived from Latin is used in words like biography meaning to write about a person's life, and biology meaning the study of living organisms.

- **Words with double meanings.** Did you know that the word husband not only means a man married to a woman, but also thrift or frugality? Sometimes, words have double meanings. The dictionary meaning, or the denotation of a word is sometimes different from the way we use it or its connotation.

- **Read widely, read deeply and read daily.** The best way to expand your vocabulary is to familiarize yourself with as many words as possible through reading. By reading, you are able to remember words in a proper context and thus, remember its meaning or at the very least, its use. Reading widely would help you get acquainted with words you may never use every day. This is the best strategy without doubt. However, if you are studying for an exam next week, or even tomorrow, it isn't much help! Below you will find a range of different ways to learn new words quickly and efficiently.

- **Remember.** Always remember the big words are easy to understand when divided into smaller parts, and the smaller words will often have several other meanings aside from the one you already know. Here are suggested effective ways to help you improve your vocabulary.

- **Be Committed To Learning New Words**. To improve your vocabulary you need to make a commitment to learn new words. Commit to learning at least a word or two a day. You can also get new words by reading books, poems, stories, plays and magazines. Expose yourself to more language to increase the number of new words that you learn.

- **Learn Practical Vocabulary**. As much as possible, learn vocabulary that is associated with what you do and that you can use regularly. For example, learn words related to your profession or hobby. Learn as much vocabulary as you can in your favorite subjects.

- **Use New Words Frequently**. When you learn a new word start using it and do so frequently. Repeat it when you are alone and try to use the word as often as you can with people you talk to. You can also use flashcards to practice new words that you learn.

- **Learn the Proper Usage.** If you do not understand the proper usage, look it up and make sure you have it right.

- **Use a Dictionary**. When reading textbooks, novels or assigned readings, keep the dictionary nearby. Also learn how to use online dictionaries and WORD dictionary. When you come across a new word, check for it's meaning. If you cannot do so immediately, then you should write it down and check it when possible. This will help you understand what the word means and exactly how best to use it.

- **Learn Word Roots, Prefixes and Suffixes.** English words are usually derived from suffixes, prefixes and roots, which come from Latin, French or Greek. Learning the root or origin of a word helps you easily understand the meaning of the word and other words that are derived from the root. Generally, if you learn the meaning of one root word, you will understand two or three words. This is a great two-for-one strategy. Most prefixes, suffixes, roots and stems are used in two, three or more words, so if you know the root, prefix or suffix, you can guess the meaning of many words.

- **Synonyms and Antonyms**. Most words in the English language have two or three (at least) synonyms and antonyms. For example, "big," in the most common usage, has seventy-five synonyms and an equal number of antonyms. Understanding the relationships between these words and how they all fit together gives your brain a framework, which makes them easier to learn, remember and recall.

- **Use Flash Cards**. Flash cards are the best way to memorize things. They can be used anywhere and anytime, so you can use odd free moments waiting for the bus or waiting in line. Make your own or buy commercially prepared flash cards, and keep them with you all the time.

- **Make word lists.** Learning vocabulary, like learning many things, requires repetition. Keep a new word journal in a separate section or separate notebook. Add any words that you look up in the dictionary, as well as from word lists. Review your word lists regularly.

Photocopying or printing off word lists from the Internet or handouts is not the same. Actually writing out the word and a few notes on the definition is an important process for imprinting the word in your brain. Writing out the word and definition in your New Word Journal, forces you to concentrate and focus on the new word. Hitting PRINT or pushing the button on the photocopier does not do the same thing.

Science

THIS SECTION CONTAINS A SCIENCE SELF-ASSESSMENT AND TUTORIALS. The tutorials are designed to familiarize students with general principles and the self-assessment contains general questions similar to the science questions likely to be on the TEAS® exam, but are not intended to be identical to the exam questions. Many Universities recommend students take an introductory Science course before taking the TEAS® Exam. The tutorials are *not* designed to be a complete science course, and it is assumed students have some familiarity with science. If you do not understand parts of the tutorial, or find the tutorial difficult, it is recommended that you seek out additional instruction.

Note that these questions are for skill practice only.

Tour of the TEAS Science Content

The TEAS® science section has 48 questions and counts for 32% of your score. Below is a detailed list of the science topics likely to appear on the TEAS®. Make sure that you understand these at the very minimum.

- Describe and understand the functions of body systems including, circulatory, digestive, nervous, respiratory and immune systems.
- Understand general human anatomy and physiology
- Birth rates, death rates and population growth
- Natural selection and adaptation
- Biological classification
- Parts of a cell and functions
- Mitosis and Meiosis
- Photosynthesis and respiration
- DNA and RNA, including mutations and cell replication
- Basic Heredity (Mendel and Punnett squares)
- Chromosomes, genes and proteins
- Phenotypes and genotypes
- Basic chemical reactions such as oxidation/reduction and acid/base reactions
- Catalysts

- Chemical bonds
- Types of energy - Kinetic, potential, mechanical
- Atoms, protons, neutrons and electrons
- The Periodic Table
- States of matter - liquids, gases and solids
- Simple changes of state including evaporation, vaporization and condensation
- Understand scientific reasoning
- Identify steps in a scientific investigation

The questions below are not the same as you will find on the TEAS® - that would be too easy! And nobody knows what the questions will be and they change all the time. Mostly the changes consist of substituting new questions for old, but the changes also can be new question formats or styles, changes to the number of questions in each section, changes to the time limits for each section and combing sections. Below are general Science questions that cover the same areas as the TEAS®. While the format and exact wording of the questions may differ slightly, and change from year to year, if you can answer the questions below, you will have no problem with the science section of the TEAS®.

Science Self Assessment

The purpose of the self-assessment is:

- Identify your strengths and weaknesses.
- Develop a personalized study plan (above)
- Get accustomed to the TEAS® format
- Extra practice – the self-assessment is a 3rd test!
- Provide a baseline score for preparing your study schedule.

Since this is a self-assessment, and depending on how confident you are with basic science, timing yourself is optional. The TEAS® has 48 science questions to be answered in 60 minutes. The self-assessment has 40 questions, so allow 50 minutes to complete.

Once complete, use the table below to assess you understanding of the content, and prepare your study schedule described in chapter 1.

80% - 100%	Excellent – you have mastered the content!
60% – 79%	Good. You have a working knowledge. Even though you can just pass this section, you may want to review the tutorials and do some extra practice to see if you can improve your mark.
40% - 59%	Below Average. You do not understand the content. Review the tutorials, and retake this quiz again in a few days, before proceeding to the practice test questions.
Less than 40%	Poor. You have a very limited understanding of the content. Please review the tutorials, and retake this quiz again in a few days, before proceeding to the practice test questions.

Science Self-Assessment Answer Sheet

1. Ⓐ Ⓑ Ⓒ Ⓓ   11. Ⓐ Ⓑ Ⓒ Ⓓ   21. Ⓐ Ⓑ Ⓒ Ⓓ
2. Ⓐ Ⓑ Ⓒ Ⓓ   12. Ⓐ Ⓑ Ⓒ Ⓓ   22. Ⓐ Ⓑ Ⓒ Ⓓ
3. Ⓐ Ⓑ Ⓒ Ⓓ   13. Ⓐ Ⓑ Ⓒ Ⓓ   23. Ⓐ Ⓑ Ⓒ Ⓓ
4. Ⓐ Ⓑ Ⓒ Ⓓ   14. Ⓐ Ⓑ Ⓒ Ⓓ   24. Ⓐ Ⓑ Ⓒ Ⓓ
5. Ⓐ Ⓑ Ⓒ Ⓓ   15. Ⓐ Ⓑ Ⓒ Ⓓ   25. Ⓐ Ⓑ Ⓒ Ⓓ
6. Ⓐ Ⓑ Ⓒ Ⓓ   16. Ⓐ Ⓑ Ⓒ Ⓓ   26. Ⓐ Ⓑ Ⓒ Ⓓ
7. Ⓐ Ⓑ Ⓒ Ⓓ   17. Ⓐ Ⓑ Ⓒ Ⓓ   27. Ⓐ Ⓑ Ⓒ Ⓓ
8. Ⓐ Ⓑ Ⓒ Ⓓ   18. Ⓐ Ⓑ Ⓒ Ⓓ   28. Ⓐ Ⓑ Ⓒ Ⓓ
9. Ⓐ Ⓑ Ⓒ Ⓓ   19. Ⓐ Ⓑ Ⓒ Ⓓ   29. Ⓐ Ⓑ Ⓒ Ⓓ
10. Ⓐ Ⓑ Ⓒ Ⓓ   20. Ⓐ Ⓑ Ⓒ Ⓓ   30. Ⓐ Ⓑ Ⓒ Ⓓ

Human Body Science

1. Which system can be thought of as the blood distribution system?

    a. Digestive system
    b. Musculoskeletal system
    c. Endocrine system
    d. Circulatory system

2. What are examples of nutrients circulated via the circulatory system?

    a. Citric acids
    b. Amino acids
    c. Proteins
    d. Nuclei

3. What is the primary purpose of the digestive system?

    a. To expel food and liquids from the body.
    b. To absorb oxygen from food.
    c. To help circulate blood throughout the body.
    d. To convert food into a form that can provide nourishment for the body.

4. Which element in the digestive process helps break down food?

    a. Digestive juices
    b. Proteins
    c. Amino acids
    d. Chromosomes

5. What is the respiratory system?

    a. The system that brings oxygen into the body and expels carbon dioxide from the body.
    b. The system that sends blood to and from the heart.
    c. The system which processes food that enters the body.
    d. The system which expels urine from the body.

Science

6. **Which, if any, of the following statements about the respiratory system are true?**

    a. The respiratory system consists of all the organs involved in breathing.

    b. Organs included in the respiratory system are the nose, pharynx, larynx, trachea, bronchi and lungs.

    c. The respiratory system conveys oxygen into our bodies and removes carbon dioxide from our bodies.

    d. All of the Above.

7. **Which of the following are an important component of the respiratory system?**

    a. The cornea
    b. The lungs
    c. The kidneys
    d. The stomach

Life Science

8. **Fill in the Blank.**

    A _____ is a naturally occurring assemblage of plants and animals that occupy a common environment.

    a. Society
    b. Biosphere
    c. Community
    d. Population

9. **Classification is a grouping of organisms based on similar**

    a. Traits and evolutionary histories
    b. Traits and biological histories
    c. Behaviors and evolutionary histories
    d. Traits and evolutionary advancement

10. **A method for categorizing organisms by their biological type is known as**

    a. Anatomical classification
    b. Biological classification
    c. Physical classification

d. Cellular classification

11. **When compared to homologous traits, "analogous" traits refer to ones that**

    a. Are similar but the similarity does not derive from a common ancestor.
    b. Are similar because they had the same parents.
    c. Are not similar and do not come from a common ancestor.
    d. Are completely equal.

12. **Which, if any, of the following statements about mitosis are correct?**

    a. Mitosis is the process of cell division by which identical daughter cells are produced.
    b. Following mitosis, new cells contain less DNA than did the original cells.
    c. During mitosis, the chromosome number is doubled.
    d. A and C are correct.

13. **What is a nucleic acid that carries the genetic information in the cell and is capable of self-replication?**

    a. RNA
    b. Triglyceride
    c. DNA
    d. DAR

14. **The segment of a DNA molecule determining the amino acid sequence of protein is known as**

    a. Operator gene
    b. Structural gene
    c. Regulator gene
    d. Modifier gene

15. **Cells that line the inner or outer surfaces of organs or body cavities are often linked together by intimate physical connections. What are these connections?**

    a. Separate desmosomes
    b. Ronofilaments
    c. Tight junctions
    d. Fascia adherenes

SCIENCE

16. Genes control heredity in man and other organisms. These genes are

    a. A segment of RNA or DNA

    b. A bead like structure on the chromosomes

    c. A protein molecule

    d. A segment of RNA

17. Describe the systems in our bodies.

    a. Our bodies have 5 different systems, including circulatory, digestive, and lymphatic.

    b. Our bodies have 11 different systems, including circulatory, digestive, and heart.

    c. Our bodies have 11 different systems, including circulatory, digestive, and lymphatic.

    d. Our bodies have 12 different systems, including circulatory, bowel, and lymphatic.

18. Who was a 19th century scientist who outlined the original theory of inheritance?

    a. Albert Einstein

    b. Christian Doppler

    c. Gregor Mendel

    d. Charles Darwin

19. Describe the science of genetics.

    a. Genetics is a branch of biology concerned with the study of heredity and variation.

    b. Genetics attempts to explain how characteristics of living organisms are passed on from one generation to the next.

    c. Genetics is a measure of the variety of the of the Earth's animal, plant, and microbial species.

    d. A and B

Earth Science

20. What is the overall measure of the variety of the Earth's animal, plant, and microbial species, of genetic differences within species, and of the ecosystems that support those species?

    a. Environment
    b. Bio-network
    c. Ecology
    d. Biodiversity

21. In the Periodic Table, elements are arranged in order of their atomic _____, which is the number of _____ found in their nucleus.

    a. Mass, protons
    b. Number, neutrons
    c. Mass, neutrons
    d. Number, protons

22. Any physical manifestation that is part of the observable structure, function or behavior of a living organism is its

    a. Genetic code
    b. Chromosome
    c. Genotype
    d. Phenotype

23. Protons, neutrons, and electrons differ in that

    a. Protons and neutrons form the nucleus of an atom, while electrons are found in fixed energy levels around the nucleus of the atom.
    b. Protons and neutrons are charged particles and electrons are neutral.
    c. Protons and neutrons form fixed energy levels around the nucleus of the atom and electrons are located near the surface of the atom.
    d. Protons, neutrons and electrons are charged particles.

SCIENCE

24. What are considered to be the four fundamental forces of nature?

    a. Gravity, electromagnetic force, weak nuclear force, and strong nuclear force

    b. Gravity, electromagnetic force, negative nuclear force, and positive nuclear force

    c. Polarity, electromagnetic force, weak nuclear force, and strong nuclear force

    d. Gravity, chemical magnetic force, weak nuclear force, and strong nuclear force

25. Which of these statements about mechanical energy is/are true?

    a. Mechanical energy is the energy that is possessed by an object due to its motion or due to its position.

    b. Mechanical energy can be either kinetic energy (energy of motion) or potential energy (stored energy of position).

    c. Objects have mechanical energy if they are in motion

    d. All of the above.

26. Evaporation is

    a. A type of vaporization that occurs within the mass of a liquid.

    b. A type of vaporization that occurs from the surface of a liquid.

    c. A type of vaporization that occurs from the surface and within the mass of a liquid.

    d. None of the above.

27. Describe enzymes.

    a. Most enzymes are proteins that are selective catalysts

    b. Enzymes are catalysts that accelerate metabolic reactions

    c. Enzymes are chemical agents that assist metabolic reactions

    d. Enzymes are biological agents that decrease the rate of reaction

Scientific Reasoning

28. In science, _____ is a difference between the desired and actual performance or behavior of a system or object.

    a. Accuracy

    b. Uncertainty

    c. Error

    d. Mistake

29. When employing the scientific method of research, the researcher follows these steps

    a. Define the question, make observations, offer a possible explanation, perform an experiment, analyze data, draw conclusions.

    b. Make observations, offer a possible explanation, define the question, perform an experiment, analyze, draw conclusions.

    c. Perform an experiment, make observations, define the question, offer a possible explanation, analyze the data, draw conclusions.

    d. Make observations, define the question, offer a possible explanation, perform an experiment, analyze data, draw conclusions.

30. What is the principle that generally advises choosing the competing hypothesis that makes the fewest new assumptions, when the hypotheses are equal in other respects?

    a. Hickam's Dictum

    b. Boyle's Law

    c. Dalton's Law

    d. Occam's Razor

SCIENCE

Answer Key

1. D
The circulatory system can be thought of as the blood distribution system.

2. B
The circulatory system is a system that passes nutrients (such as amino acids, electrolytes and lymph), gases, hormones, blood cells, etc. to and from cells in the body to help fight diseases, help stabilize body temperature and pH.

3. D
The primary purpose of the digestive system is to convert food into a form that can provide nourishment for the body.

4. A
Digestive juices such as gastric acid are formed in the stomach. It has a pH of 1 to 2 and is composed of hydrochloric acid (HCl) (around 0.5%, or 5000 parts per million), and large quantities of potassium chloride (KCl) and sodium chloride (NaCl). The acid plays a key role in digestion of proteins, by activating digestive enzymes, and making ingested proteins unravel so that digestive enzymes can break down the long chains of amino acids.

5. A
The respiratory system is the anatomical system of an organism that introduces respiratory gases to the interior and performs gas exchange. The anatomical features of the respiratory system include airways, lungs, and the respiratory muscles. Molecules of oxygen and carbon dioxide are passively exchanged, by diffusion, between the gaseous external environment and the blood. This exchange process occurs in the alveolar region of the lungs.

6. D
All the statements are true.

   a. The respiratory system consists of all the organs involved in breathing.

   b. Organs included in the respiratory system are the nose, pharynx, larynx, trachea, bronchi and lungs.

   c. The respiratory system conveys oxygen into our bodies and removes carbon dioxide from our bodies.

7. B
The Lungs are an important component of the respiratory system.

8. C
Communities are usually named after a dominant feature, such as characteristic plant species, e.g., pine.

9. A
Classification is a grouping of organisms based on similar traits and evolutionary histories.

Note: Taxonomy and systematics are the two sciences that attempt to classify living things. In taxonomy, organisms are assigned to groups based on their characteristics. In modern systematics, the placement of organisms into groups is based on evolutionary relationships.

10. B
Biological classification. Classification is more a matter of convenience; in reality, there are many times when the various classifications tend to blur.

11 A
Analogous traits are similar but the similarity does not derive from a common ancestor.

12. D
A and C are correct.

> a. Mitosis is the process of cell division by which identical daughter cells are produced.
>
> c. During mitosis, the chromosome number is doubled.

13. C
DNA is a nucleic acid that carries the genetic information in the cell and is capable of self-replication.

14. B
A structural gene is the segment of a DNA molecule determining the amino acid sequence of protein. DNA is a nucleic acid that contains the genetic instructions used in the development and functioning of all known living organisms (except for RNA viruses). The DNA segments that carry this genetic information are called genes but other DNA sequences have structural purposes or are involved in regulating the use of this genetic information. Along with RNA and proteins DNA is one of the three major macromolecules that are essential for all known forms of life. [3]

15. C
Tight junctions or zonula occludens are the closely associated areas of two cells whose membranes join forming a virtually impermeable barrier to fluid. It is a type of junctional complex present only in vertebrates. The corresponding junctions that occur in invertebrates are septate junctions. [4]

16. A
Genes are made from a long molecule called DNA which is copied and inherited across generations. DNA is made of simple units that line up in a particular order within this large molecule. The order of these units carries genetic information similar to how the order of letters on a page carries information. The language used by DNA is called the genetic code which lets organisms read the information in the genes. This information is

the instruction for constructing and operating a living organism.

17. C
Our bodies have 11 different systems, including circulatory, digestive, and lymphatic.

Note: Other systems include the endocrine, immune, muscular, nervous, reproductive, respiratory, skeletal, and urinary systems.

18. C
Gregor Mendel was a 19th century scientist who outlined the original theory of inheritance.

19. D
    a. Is a branch of biology concerned with the study of heredity and variation.

    b. Attempts to explain how characteristics of living organisms are passed on from one generation to the next.

20. D
Biodiversity is an overall measure of the variety of the Earth's animal, plant, and microbial species, of genetic differences within species, and of the ecosystems that support those species.

Note: In the 20th century, the destruction of the rainforests and the spread of agriculture is believed to have resulted in the most severe and rapid loss of diversity in the history of the planet.

21. D
In the Periodic Table, elements are arranged in order of their atomic number, which is the number of protons found in their nucleus.

22. D
Any physical manifestation that is part of the observable structure, function or behavior of a living organism is its phenotype.

23. A
Protons and neutrons form the nucleus of an atom, while electrons are found infixed energy levels around the nucleus of the atom.

24. A
The four fundamental forces of nature are, gravity, electromagnetic force, weak nuclear force, and strong nuclear force.

Note: Electromagnetic force is more commonly known as electricity.

25. D
All the statements are true.

a. Mechanical energy is the energy possessed by an object due to its motion or due to its position.

b. Mechanical energy can be either kinetic energy (energy of motion) or potential energy (stored energy of position).

c. Objects have mechanical energy if they are in motion

26. B
Evaporation is a type of vaporization of a liquid that only occurs on the surface of a liquid. The other type of vaporization is boiling, which, instead, occurs within the entire mass of the liquid.

27. A
Most enzymes are proteins that are selective catalysts.

28. C
In science, Error is a difference between the desired and actual performance or behavior of a system or object.

29. A
When employing the scientific method of research, the researcher follows these steps: define the question, make observations, offer a possible explanation, perform an experiment, analyze data, draw conclusions.

30. D
Occam's Razor is a principle that generally advises choosing the competing hypothesis that makes the fewest new assumptions, when the hypotheses are equal in other respects.

Science Tutorials

Scientific Method

The scientific method is a set of steps that allow people who ask "how" and "why" questions about the world to go about finding valid answers that accurately reflect reality.

> Were it not for the scientific method, people would have no valid method for drawing quantifiable and accurate information about the world.

SCIENCE

There are four primary steps to the scientific method:

1. Analyzing an aspect of reality and asking "how" or "why" it works or exists
2. Forming a hypothesis that explains "how" or "why"
3. Making a prediction about the sort of things that would happen if the hypothesis were true
4. Performing an experiment to test your prediction.

These steps vary somewhat depending on the field of science you happen to be studying. (In astronomy, for instance, experiments are generally eschewed in favor of observational evidence confirming that predictions are true.) But for the most part, this is the model scientists follow.

Observation and Analysis

The first step in the scientific method requires you to determine what it is about reality that you want to explore.

You might notice that your friends who eat regular servings of fruits and vegetables are healthier and more athletic than your friends who live off red meat and meals covered in cheese and gravy. This is an observation and, noting it, you are likely to ask yourself "why" it seems to be true. At this stage of the scientific method, scientists will often do research to see if anyone else has explored similar observations and analyze what other people's findings have been. This is an important step not only because shows what others have found to be true about their observation, but because it can show what others have found to be false, which can be equally valuable.

Hypothesis

After making your observation and doing some research, you can form your hypothesis. A hypothesis is an idea you formulate based on the evidence you have already gathered about "how" your observation relates to reality.

Using the example of your friends' diets, you may have found research discussing vitamin levels in fruits and vegetables and how certain vitamins will affect a person's health and athleticism. This research may lead you to hypothesize that the foods your healthy friends are eating contain specific types of vitamins, and it is the vitamins making them healthy. Just as importantly, however, is applying research that shows hypotheses that were later proven wrong. Scientists need to know this information, too, as it can help keep them from making errors in their thinking. For instance, you could come across a research paper in which someone hypothesized that the sugars in fruits and vegetables gave people more energy, which then helped them be more athletic. If the paper were to go onto explain that no such link was found, and that the protein and carbohydrates in meat and gravy contained far more energy than the sugar, you would know that this hypothesis was wrong and that there was no need for you to waste time exploring it.

Prediction

The third step in the scientific method is making a prediction based on your hypothesis.

Forming predictions is vital to the scientific method, because, if your prediction turns out to be correct, it will demonstrate that your hypothesis can accurately explain some aspect of the world. This is important because one aspect of the scientific method is its ability to prove objectively that your way of understanding the world is valid. We can take the simple example of a car that will not start. If you notice the fuel gauge is pointing towards empty, you can announce your prediction to the other passengers that a careful test of the gas tank will show the car has no fuel. While this seems obvious, it is still important to note since a prediction like this is the only way to really *prove* to your friends that you understand how a fuel gauge works and what it means.

In the same way a prediction made by a hypothesis is the only way to really show that it represents reality. For instance, based on your vitamin hypothesis you may predict people can be healthy and athletic while eating whatever they want as long as they take vitamin supplements. If this prediction ends being true, it will show that it is in fact the vitamins, and only the vitamins, in fruits and vegetables that make people healthy and athletic. It will prove that your hypothesis shows how vitamins work.

Experiment

The final step is to perform an experiment that tests your prediction.

You may decide to separate your healthy friends into three groups, give one group vitamin supplements and prohibit them from eating vegetables, give another fake supplements and prohibit them from eating vegetables and have the third act normally as the control group. It is always important to have a control group so you have someone acting "normally" to compare your results against. If this experiment shows the real supplement group and the control group maintaining the same level of health and athleticism while the fake supplement group grows weak and sickly, you will know your hypothesis is true. If, on the other hand, you get unexpected results, you will need to go back to step one, analyze your results, make new observations and try again with a different hypothesis.

Any hypothesis that cannot be confirmed with experiment (or in the case of fields such as astronomy, with observation) cannot be considered true and must be altered or abandoned. It is in this stage where scientists—being humans, with human beliefs and prejudices—are most likely to abandon the scientific method. If an experiment or observation gives a scientist results that he or she does not like, the scientist may be inclined to ignore the results rather than reexamine the hypothesis. This was the case for nearly a thousand years in astronomy with astronomers attempting to form accurate models of the solar system based on circular orbits of the planets and on Earth being in the center. For philosophical reasons it was believed that circles were "perfect" and that the Earth was "important," so no model that had the correct elliptical orbits or the sun properly in the center was accepted until the 16th century, even though those models more accurately described all astronomers' observations.

Cell Biology

Cell biology (formerly cytology, from the Greek kytos, "contain") is a scientific discipline that studies cells – their physiological properties, their structure, the organelles they contain, interactions with their environment, their life cycle, division and death.

>This is done both on a microscopic and molecular level. Cell biology research encompasses both the great diversity of single-celled organisms like bacteria and protozoa, as well as the many specialized cells in multicellular organisms such as humans.

Knowing the components of cells and how cells work is fundamental to all biological sciences.

>Appreciating the similarities and differences between cell types is particularly important to the fields of cell and molecular biology as well as to biomedical fields such as cancer research and developmental biology. These fundamental similarities and differences provide a unifying theme, sometimes allowing the principles learned from studying one cell type to be extrapolated and generalized to other cell types. Therefore, research in cell biology is closely related to genetics, biochemistry, molecular biology, immunology, and developmental biology.

Each type of protein is usually sent to a particular part of the cell.

>An important part of cell biology is the investigation of molecular mechanisms by which proteins are moved to different places inside cells or secreted from cells.

Processes – Movement of Proteins

Most proteins are synthesized by ribosomes in the rough endoplasmic reticulum.

>Ribosomes contain the nucleic acid RNA, which assembles and joins amino acids to make proteins. They can be found alone or in groups within the cytoplasm as well as on the RER.

This process is known as protein biosynthesis.

>Biosynthesis (also called biogenesis) is an enzyme-catalyzed process in cells of living organisms by which substrates are converted to more complex products (also simply known as protein translation). Some proteins, such as those to be incorporated in membranes (known as membrane proteins), are transported into the "rough" endoplasmic reticulum (ER) during synthesis. This process can be

followed by transportation and processing in the Golgi apparatus.

The Golgi apparatus is a large organelle that processes proteins and prepares them for use both inside and outside the cell.

The Golgi apparatus is somewhat like a post office. It receives items (proteins from the ER), packages and labels them, and then sends them on to their destinations (to different parts of the cell or to the cell membrane for transport out of the cell). From the Golgi, membrane proteins can move to the plasma membrane, to other sub-cellular compartments, or they can be secreted from the cell.

The ER and Golgi can be thought of as the "membrane protein synthesis compartment" and the "membrane protein processing compartment", respectively.

There is a semi-constant flux of proteins through these compartments. ER and Golgi-resident proteins associate with other proteins but remain in their respective compartments. Other proteins "flow" through the ER and Golgi to the plasma membrane. Motor proteins transport membrane protein-containing vesicles along cytoskeletal tracks to distant parts of cells such as axon terminals.

Some proteins that are made in the cytoplasm contain structural features that target them for transport into mitochondria or the nucleus.

Some mitochondrial proteins are made inside mitochondria and are coded for by mitochondrial DNA. In plants, chloroplasts also make some cell proteins.

Extracellular and cell surface proteins destined to be degraded can move back into intracellular compartments upon being incorporated into endocytosed vesicles some of which fuse with lysosomes where the proteins are broken down to their individual amino acids. The degradation of some membrane proteins begins while still at the cell surface when they are separated by secretases. Proteins that function in the cytoplasm are often degraded by proteasomes.

SCIENCE

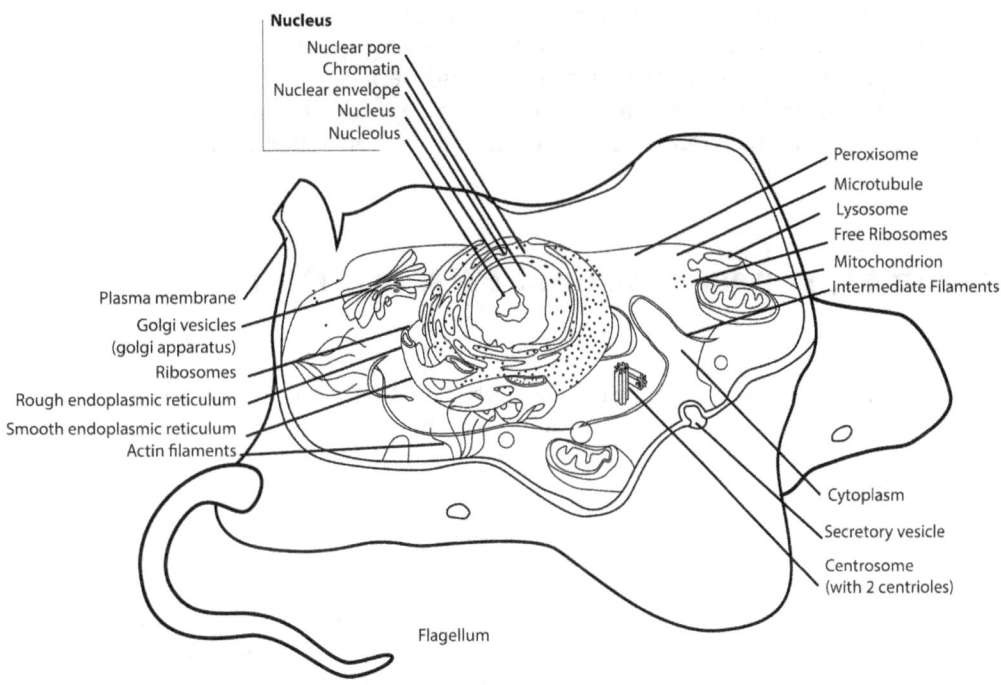

Other cellular processes

Active and Passive transport - Movement of molecules into and out of cells.
Autophagy - The process whereby cells "eat" their own internal components or microbial invaders.
Adhesion - Holding together cells and tissues.
Reproduction - Made possible by the combination of sperm made in the testiculi (contained in some male cells' nuclei) and the egg made in the ovary (contained in the nucleus of a female cell). When the sperm breaks through the hard outer shell of the egg a new cell embryo is formed, which, in humans, grows to full size in 9 months.
Cell movement - Chemotaxis, Contraction, cilia and flagella.
Cell signalling - Regulation of cell behavior by signals from outside.
DNA repair and Cell death
Metabolism - Glycolysis, respiration, Photosynthesis
Transcription and mRNA splicing - gene expression.**Internal cellular structures**

Cytoplasm - contents of the main fluid-filled space inside cells
Chloroplast - organelle for photosynthesis
Cilia - motile microtubule containing structures of eukaryotes

Cytoskeleton - protein filaments
Endoplasmic reticulum - major site of protein synthesis
Golgi apparatus - site of protein glycosylation in the endomembrane system
Flagella - motile structures of bacteria, archaea and eukaryotes
Lysosome - breaks down cellular waste products and debris
Nucleus - holds DNA of eukaryotic cells and controls cellular activities
Ribosome - RNA and protein complex required for protein synthesis in cells

Chromosomes, genes, proteins, RNA and DNA

The concepts of genes, chromosomes, proteins, RNA and DNA are all interrelated genetic terms. Chromosomes are made up of genes, the DNA contains the chromosomes and the RNA interprets and implements the information in the RNA. Here is a break down of each of them.

Proteins

Proteins are biological molecules that are made up of a chain or chains of amino acids. Proteins play many very vital roles in living organisms. Protein is essential for the performance of many bodily functions such as replicating DNA, transporting nutrients and molecules within the body, responding to stimuli, and acting as a catalyst for metabolic reactions within the living organism, among other things. There are different types of proteins and they play various roles. The difference in proteins would be determined by their unique arrangement or sequence of amino acids.

Genes

A gene is the molecular hereditary unity of an organism and a small part of the chromosome. It is the term used to describe a portion of RNA or DNA code that performs a particular function in the organism. Genes are essential to life because they specify the functions of all proteins and RNA chains. Genes contain the information to maintain and build the cells in the organism and also contain genetic information that would be passed onto the offspring.

Genes hold the information for biological traits and functions some of which can clearly be seen and some of which are hidden. For example, the information contained in specific genes determines factors such as eye color, hair color, number of limbs, height and so on. Some traits such as blood type and the thousands of metabolic reactions and biochemical process that take place in the body to sustain life are defined unseen by the genes.

A gene is set of basic instruction embedded on a sequence of nucleic acids. The gene is a locatable region of the DNA genome sequence that correspond to a unit of inheritance and associated with a particular body function or set of functions.

Chromosomes

The chromosome is a piece of the DNA containing several genes. The chromosome is an organized part of the DNA. It is a single piece of coiled DNA. The chromosome contains several genes, DNA-bound proteins, nucleotide sequences and regulatory elements. The DNA-bound proteins help to hold the DNA together and regulate its functions.

Since the chromosomes contain the genes, they contain almost all the genetic information of the organism. Chromosomes differ from one organism to another. The DNA molecule could be linear or circular. The chromosome can contain from 100,000 to over 3 million nucleotides in one long chain depending on the organism. Cells with defined nuclei (eukaryotic cells) usually have large linear shaped chromosomes. Cells without clearly defined nuclei (prokaryotic cells) usually have smaller sized circular chromosomes.

Chromosomes are essential in the process of cell division. In mitosis cell division, the chromosomes have to be replicated and then divided among the two resulting daughter cells. This ensures that the resulting two daughter cells are genetically identical to the original mother cell.

DNA

DNA or Deoxyribonucleic acid is an essential component of life. It has been described as the blueprint of a living organism. It contains vital genetic information and instructions that are required for the proper functioning and development of all types and forms of living organisms and even viruses. DNA, proteins and RNA are the three most important macro-molecules that are essential for any form of life.

The genetic information contained in the DNA is encoded as a sequence of nucleotides known as G, A, and C. With G being guanine, A, adenine, T, thymine and C cytosine. These nucleotides are arranged as DNA molecules in a double-stranded helix. The strands run in opposite directions and are thus anti-parallel. The DNA contains long structures known as chromosomes.

RNA

RNA or Ribonucleic acids are large biological molecules that perform the important roles of decoding, coding, regulating and expressing the genes and the information contained within them. RNA, DNA and proteins are three essential components for all form of life. The RNA is also composed of nucleotides, but unlike the DNA that is double stranded, the RNA is single stranded.

In organisms, some RNA components serve as messengers to convey genetic information to direct the synthesis or use of specific proteins for specific purposes. It can thus be said that RNA is essential for the proper carrying out of the information contained in the DNA genes. RNA plays important roles within the cell such as helping to catalyze biological reactions sense and communicate cellular signals and control gene expressions. RNA is also essential for protein synthesis.

Mitosis and Meiosis

Meiosis and mitosis are two types of cellular division and they play a very important role in cell reproduction and the maintenance of tissues.

The cell is the basic functional unit of living organisms. It is made up of a collection of organelles and other cell matter dispersed within the cell membrane. For new cells to form, existing cells divide through the process of meiosis or mitosis, depending on the type of cell and reason for division.

Mitosis refers to the division of a cell into two identical cells.

The original cell goes through a process of duplication of its genetic material and then equally divides its contents into two new daughter cells. The process of mitosis goes through several stages until the two cells segregate to form two distinct but genetically identical cells.

Mitosis cell division

During mitosis the cell divides its nucleus and then separates its organelles and chromosomes into two identical parts. The mother cell then divides into two genetically identical cells with equal parts of the cellular contents. The nuclei, cell membrane, organelles and cytoplasm of the cell would be shared between the two new cells.

Mitosis cell division is a complex and fast process. The process takes place in stages with each stage comprising of a set of activities that leads to the next set. The stages of mitosis are Prophase, Prometaphase, Metaphase, Anaphase and Telophase. Mitosis occurs in some unicellular organisms and within animal and human cells. Unicellular organisms use mitosis to reproduce their like and within animal and humans, mitosis is used to replace cells and repair tissues.

SCIENCE

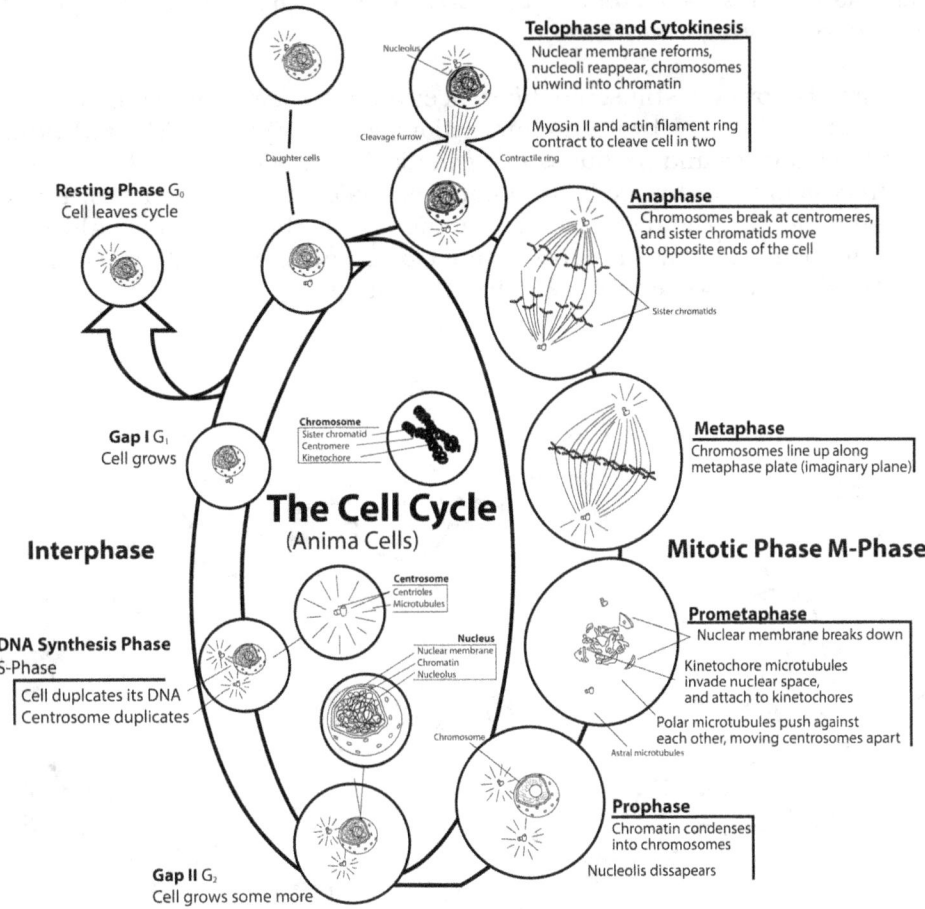

Meiosis

Meiosis occurs when one cells from the male and female combines or fuses together to form one diploid cell, which then splits to form four haploid cells.

The diploid cell contains copies of the chromosome and genetic information from both parents. The resulting four haploid cells will contain a copy of each chromosome.

Each chromosome in the four cells will contain a unique blend of the paternal and maternal genetic information, which makes it possible for the offspring to share some genetic resemblance to both parents while remaining genetically distinct from both of them. This nature of meiosis cell division is what accounts for the genetic diversity that is available today as each offspring DNA is a unique blend of its maternal and paternal genetic DNA.

Mitosis and meiosis have some similarities in that they are both types of cell division among living organisms.

There is however still some differences among them. For example, mitosis occurs within a cell with no interactions with other cells. The individual cell simply divides and produces two genetically identical cells. With meiosis, the process involves two cells from both the male and female in a form sexual reproduction. The resultant cells are four cells that are genetically different from their parents. The process of meiosis was discovered by Oscar Hertwig and Mitosis was discovered by Walther Flemming.

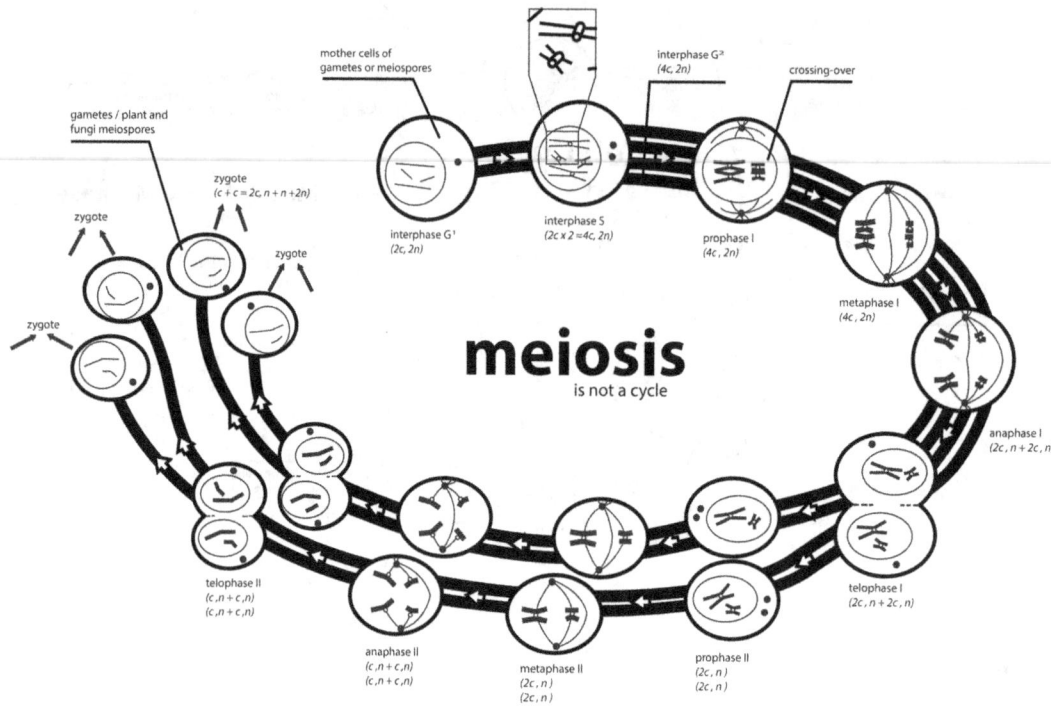

Phenotypes and Genotypes

The terms "phenotype" and "genotype" were first introduced in 1911 by Wilhelm Johannsen.

The term genotype refers to the genes of an organism that contains its complete hereditary information.
Phenotype refers to the actual observed properties of the organism.

Phenotypes deal with morphology, behavior and development. The distinction between genotypes and phenotypes is a very important fundamental aspect in the study of hereditary traits.

To explain the differences between the two concepts, one may look at genotypes as the inherited information about an organism. It is the genetic makeup of the traits, features and characteristics of the organism. Phenotype on the other hand defines the way that the information as spelled out by the genes is represented. Phenotype deals with the actual observable development and behavior.

A small or even minute difference in the genes of two organisms would mean that the two organisms have different genotypes.

Genes are hereditary and the genetic information contained is passed down from parents under control of specific molecular mechanisms. The genes or genetic information therein contained would affect or control the representation of the phenotype.

The genes define the trait or feature of the organism while the phenotype is the observable demonstration or expression of that trait. For example, if a mouse has a white color, it can be said that the genes defines that the mouse would be white and the phenotype is the white color that is observable. The genotype determines the phenotype, but the phenotype is also affected by external factors such as environmental factors.

A set of genotypes mapped to a set of phenotypes are referred to as a genotype-phenotype map.

The genotype is the largest influencer of an organism's phenotype, but is not the only influencing factor. That is why two identical twins that share the same genotype would still not have the same phenotypes. They may share identical genomes and their phenotype may even be quit similar, but it cannot be the same. That is why parents and close fiends would always be able to tell them apart. This is because their phenotype or the representation or expression of their genetic makeup as contained in their genotype would not be the same.

The term phenotype plasticity is used to describe the extent to which the genotype of an organism determines its phenotype.

An organism with weak or little phenotype plasticity would be highly determined more by its genotype and less by environmental factors.

An organism with high phenotype plasticity would have its phenotype more affected by environmental factors than by its genotype. A good example of an organism with high plasticity whose phenotype is more dependant on its environment than its genotype is the larval newt. The larvae would grow larger sized tails and heads relative to their body size when it notices the presence of their natural predators, i.e., the dragonfly.

Phenotype canalization is a term used to describe the extent that an organism's phenotype can be used to draw conclusions about the organism's genotype.

An organism with a canalized phenotype would be rarely affected by changes in its genotypes. If canalization is absent, very minor changes in the genome would result in immediate changes in the resulting phenotype.

Heredity: Genes and Mutation

All of the genetic material that tells our cells what jobs they hold is stored in our DNA (deoxyribonucleic acid). When complex creatures such as humans reproduce, our DNA is copied and combined with our mate's DNA to create a new genetic sequence for our offspring.

This information is stored in our genes and encoded in DNA base pairs through different combinations of the chemical groupings adenine and thymine (represented by A and T) and guanine and cytosine (represented by G and C). Each gene covers a small portion of our DNA and is responsible for creating the protein that section of DNA holds instructions for.

Genes contain two alleles, one from each of our parents. When we reproduce we will transfer one, and only one, of each allele to our children.

Alleles can be either dominant or recessive, and by combining the pairs of alleles we get from our parents, we can determine what our genes say we should be like. This genetic description of ourselves is known as our genotype. Genotype is our exact genetic makeup, and it determines our physical characteristics such as basic hair, eye and skin color. Related to the genotype is our phenotype, which describes the characteristics we display when our genes interact with the environment. For example, skin color is determined by a person's genotype, but the effect the sun has on skin—does the person tan, freckle, bun or even come away without any noticeable effect at all?—is an expression of phenotype.

Under normal circumstances people's genes will transfer directly from their parents following Mendel's Laws of Inheritance. Errors are common though.

DNA reproduction, however, is not necessarily a flawless process. Errors can develop either at random or due to outside influences such as radiation or chemicals in the environment. These errors, when related to heredity are called de novo mutations; they occur during embryonic development. Some mutations have no effect at all on the person's genetic makeup, but others can alter the way genes express themselves. Whether this is a good thing or not depends entirely on what genes are altered in what ways. Some mutations can cause children to be born sick or to have a higher susceptibility to disease by changing the types of proteins that their genes produce, or even by stopping certain proteins from being produced all together. Others, though, can be an improvement to the child's genetic structure. It is important to remember that the entire process of evolution is based on how random mutations throughout history have affected an individual's ability to interact with the environment.

Several notable examples of beneficial mutations stemming from natural selection can be seen in bubonic plague resistant European populations and malaria resistant African populations.

Both groups have genes built from specific alleles that create disease blocking proteins. (The CCR5 protein in people of European descent blocks the plague—and HIV sometimes—and the sickle cell protein in people of African descent blocks malaria.) These genes are widespread throughout their respective populations as a result of natural selection, which killed those who lived in these groups' ancestral regions but who did not possess the mutation. Had these diseases never existed, the mutations would have been considered neutral, providing no benefit yet causing no harm.

There are several ways that errors in DNA reproduction can cause mutations.

Chemicals can be inserted into, or deleted from base pairs, causing the chemical composition of the pairs to change and, thus, changing the alleles of the gene represented by those pairs. A portion of the DNA strand may also duplicate itself, or it may shift itself, causing the half of the base pair on one side of the DNA strand to link to the wrong half on the other side.

Heredity: Mendelian Inheritance

The father of genetics was a 19th century Austrian monk named Gregor Johann Mendel who became famous for his work crossbreeding peas in the garden of his monastery.

Aside from his life as a monk, Mendel was a highly educated physicist, studying first at the University of Olomouc (in the modern day Czech Republic) and later at the University of Vienna.

Mendel's work with peas revolutionized the scientific understanding of heredity and yielded two important laws: the Law of Segregation and the Law of Independent Assortment. To better understand these laws, however, we first need to look at the work of another geneticist, Reginald Punnett.

In 1900 while Punnett was doing his graduate work at the University of Cambridge in England, Gregor Mendel's work on genetics, which did not receive much attention during his lifetime, was being rediscovered. Punnett became an early follower of Mendelian genetics and developed the Punnett square as a means to organize the assortment of inherited alleles as Mendel described them. A Punnett square is simply a box with several squares drawn inside it and with the allele for a particular gene from each parent listed on either the top or the side. Each square shows a possible genotype (or set of alleles that define the gene) that can be inherited by the offspring of those parents. We will see Punnett squares as we explain Mendel's laws.

Law of Segregation

Mendel's Law of Segregation says that only half of the alleles of each parent's genes are transferred to their offspring, with the other half coming from the other parent.

Each gene contains two alleles. For instance a gene for trait 'A' could contain the alleles AA, Aa or aa, with the 'A' being the dominant form of the allele and 'a' being the recessive form. (Offspring with one or more dominant alleles exhibit the trait; offspring with only recessive forms do not.) The Law of Segregation says that one allele will come from one parent, and one will come from the other, and it is the parent's combined genetic makeup (rather than one parents particular genotype) that will determine the genes of their offspring.

Mendel also showed that the probability a certain trait would spread from parents to children was 3:1, if both parents had one dominant and one recessive form of the gene, also known has having heterozygous alleles. (Having two of the same alleles—AA or aa—is homozygous.)

Punnett squares

The Punnett square below represents the possible children born to two parents with Aa alleles expressing the 'A' gene.

	A	a
A	**AA**	**Aa**
a	**Aa**	aa

The three genes in bold, with at least one capital letter (AA, Aa and the other Aa), represent cases in which the presence of at least one dominant allele will cause the trait to manifest in the offspring. The remaining one (aa) represents the one case where the child does not manifest the trait even though both his or her parents do. (This could be the one brunette in a family of redheads, for instance.) Provided both parents have one dominant and one recessive allele, the distribution will always be 3:1.

Law of Independent Assortment

Mendel's second law, the Law of Independent Assortment, shows that the alleles of multiple genes will mix independently.

When two separate genotypes are tracked, the genes will produce 16 separate possible combinations spread out in a 9:3:3:1 ratio. This is also known as a dihybrid cross, while dealing with a single set of alleles is a monohybrid cross.

We can demonstrate this by assuming that we have a male and a female each with heterozygous alleles making them blond and tall. We can represent this with the genotypes BbTt in each. We should also assume that a 'bb' genotype would give someone brown hair and 'tt' would make them short. Since the Law of Independent Assortment says that each allele will mix independently, we end with four combinations of genotype that each parent can pass on: BT, Bt, bT and bt. These can then be mapped in a slightly larger Punnett square that looks like this:

	BT	Bt	bT	bt
BT	**BBTT**	**BBTt**	**BbTT**	**BbTt**
Bt	**BBTt**	BBtt	**BbTt**	Bbtt
bT	**BbTT**	**BbTt**	bbTT	bbTt
bt	**BbTt**	Bbtt	bbTt	bbtt

This is the distribution of the tall, blond couple's possible children. Nine would also be tall and blond, three would be short and blond, three would be tall and brunette, and one would be short and brunette. This perfectly follows the 9:3:3:1 ratio set out by Mendel.

Classification

Classification

Taxonomic classification is the primary method of organizing the Earth's biology. Taxonomy means,

1. The classification of organisms in an ordered system that indicates natural relationships.
2. The science, laws, or principles of classification

> The earliest form of classification that bears any resemblance to the current system can be traced back to ancient Greece with Aristotle's organization of animals based on reproduction.

The classification into kingdoms (animal, mineral and vegetable) was developed by Carolus Linnaeus.

> The true father of modern taxonomical classification, however, is Carolus Linnaeus, who in the early 18th century developed a system of kingdoms that separated life into the categories animal, mineral and vegetable. Although Linnaeus's work lacked what would today be considered essential technologies (such as microscopes capable of imaging bacteria) and theories (such as evolution), much of his system has survived in modern classification.

Charles Darwin's theory of evolution was an important factor in taxonomic classification.

With Charles Darwin's publication of On the Origin of Species in 1859 the evolutionary process became a major factor in taxonomic classification. For the first time biology could be classified by grouping the direct descendents of common ancestors rather than just grouping creatures with similar characteristics.

The main classifications are, domain, kingdom, phylum, class, order, family, genus and species.

Today, most scientists accept a hierarchical structuring of biology that goes from general, or large, to specific: domain, kingdom, phylum, class, order, family, genus and species. (There are sometimes smaller subcategories such as superfamily, subfamily, tribe and subspecies listed, but these are the primary eight categories.) Domain is the newest of these and is split into three primary groups: Bacteria, Archaea and Eukarya.
Each of these domains is split again with Bacteria splitting into the Kingdom Bacteria, Archaea splitting into the Kingdom Archaea and Eukarya splitting into the four kingdoms of Protista, Plantae, Fungi and finally our kingdom, Animalia. The Domain Eukarya splits so many times because eukaryotic cells are highly complex, containing such important features as cell walls and nuclei. As a result of this complexity, eukaryotic cells have gone through a much more diverse evolutionary process than prokaryotic cells such as bacteria and archaea, and thus Eukarya make up all complex life on Earth.

Each Kingdom has a huge number of organisms. Bacteria and Archaea (single celled organisms).

Within each of the kingdoms the number of creatures is far too many to list. It is estimated that there could be as many as 100 million different species on Earth, although nowhere near that many have been physically catalogued. Of these, the majority are Bacteria and Archaea.

Another Example - Homo Sapiens

Since there is no way to list all the different subdivisions of life on Earth here, we might as well focus on one specific animal: us, Homo sapiens. We are members of the Domain Eukarya, the Kingdom Animalia, the Phylum Chordata, the Class Mammalia, the Order Primates, the Family Hominidae, the Genus Homo, the Species Homo sapiens and finally the Subspecies Homo sapiens sapiens. This classification is able to demonstrate our exact biological position in relation to life on Earth.

One important thing, a system like this tells us is that Homo, which is Latin for "human," is not actually our species, but our genus. This is an easy fact to forget since we are currently the only member of our genus not yet extinct.

But anthropologically speaking there have been many humans including Homo habilis, Homo erectus and Homo neanderthalensis.

Taxonomical classification is an evolutionary map

Furthermore, the taxonomical classification system can be seen as a map of evolution on the planet. Plants, animals and bacteria can be traced back to common ancestors and newly discovered species can be classified in relation to their ancestors, descendants and cousins. The Genus Homo, for instance, is a direct offshoot of the Tribe Hominini. (A tribe is a subcategory of the category of family, which here is Hominidae.) Another genus that falls under the Tribe Hominini is Pan, which houses the species Chimpanzee. This shows us that until relatively recently in the history of life, Homo sapiens and Chimpanzees were the same creature, and that Chimpanzees only split off just before Homo sapiens became fully human.

Basic Chemistry

Chemistry is the science of matter, especially its chemical reactions, but also its composition, structure and properties. Chemistry is concerned with atoms and their interactions with other atoms, and particularly with the properties of chemical bonds.

Chemistry is sometimes called "the central science" because it connects physics with other natural sciences such as geology and biology. Chemistry is a branch of physical science but distinct from physics.

Traditional chemistry starts with the study of elementary particles, atoms, molecules, substances, metals, crystals and other aggregates of matter. in solid, liquid, and gas states, whether in isolation or combination. The interactions, reactions and transformations that are studied in chemistry are a result of interaction either between different chemical substances or between matter and energy.

A chemical reaction is a transformation of some substances into one or more different substances.

It can be symbolically depicted through a chemical equation. The number of atoms on the left and the right in the equation for a chemical transformation is most often equal. The nature of chemical reactions a substance may undergo and the energy changes that may accompany it are constrained by certain basic rules, known as chemical laws.

Energy and entropy considerations are invariably important in almost all chemical studies.

Chemical substances are classified in terms of their structure, phase as well as their chemical compositions. They can be analyzed using the tools of chemical analysis, e.g. spectroscopy and chromatography. Scientists engaged in chemical research are known as chemists. Most chemists specialize in one or more sub-disciplines.

Basic Concepts in Chemistry

Atoms

Atoms are some of the basic building blocks of matter. Each atom is an element—an identifiable substance that cannot be further broken down into other identifiable substances.

There are just over 100 such elements, and each of them can combine with themselves and with other elements to create all the various molecules that exist in the universe. The poison gas chlorine and the explosive metal sodium, for instance, can combine at the atomic level to form sodium chloride, also known as salt.

For thousands of years atoms were thought to be the smallest thing possible. (The word "atom" comes from an ancient Greek word meaning "unbreakable.") However, experiments performed in the mid to late 19th century began to show the presence of small particles, electrons, in electric current. By the early 20th century, the electron was known to be a part of the atom that orbited a yet undefined atomic core. A few years later, in 1919, the proton was discovered and found to exist in the nuclei of all atoms.

The protons and neutrons inside an atomic nucleus are not fundamental particles. That is, they can be divided into still smaller pieces.

Protons and neutrons are known as hadrons, which is a class of particle made up of quarks. (Quarks are a fundamental particle.) There are two distinct types of hadrons, baryons and mesons, and both protons and neutrons are baryons, meaning they are both made up of a combination of three quarks. Besides being hadrons, protons and neutrons are also known as nucleons because of their place within the nucleus. Protons have a mass of around 1.6726×10^{-27} kg and neutrons have a nearly identical mass of 1.6929×10^{-27} kg. Both particles have a ½ spin.

The number of protons inside an atomic nucleus determines what element the atom is.

An element with only one proton, for instance, is hydrogen. An element with two is helium. One with three is lithium, and so on. No element (except for hydrogen) can exist with only protons in its nucleus. Atoms need neutrons to bond the protons together using the strong force. In general atoms (again except for hydrogen) have an equal number of protons and neutrons in their nuclei.

SCIENCE

Atoms with an uneven number of protons and neutrons are called isotopes.

Isotopes have all the same chemical properties as their evenly balanced counterparts, but their nuclei are not usually as stable and are more willing to react with other elements. (Two deuterium atoms, hydrogen isotopes with one proton and one neutron in their nucleus rather than only one proton, will fuse much more readily than two regular hydrogen atoms.)

Nearly all of an atoms' mass is within its nucleus. Outside that there is a lot of empty space occupied only by a few, tiny electrons.

Electrons were once viewed as orbiting an atom like planets orbit the sun. We now know that this is wrong in several ways. For one, electrons do not really "orbit" in the sense we are used to. At the quantum level no particle is really a particle, but is actually both a particle and a wave simultaneously. Heisenberg's uncertainty principle looks at this odd truth about reality and says that you can never watch an electron orbit the nucleus as you would watch the Earth orbit the sun. Instead, you have to observe only one of the electron's physical characteristics at a time, either viewing it as a particle in a fixed position outside the nucleus or as a wave encircling the nucleus like a halo.
Additionally, planets orbiting their stars can orbit at any distance they want. In fact, every object in our solar system has an elliptical orbit, meaning that they all move in more oval rather than circular shapes, getting closer and farther from the sun at various points. Electrons cannot do this under any circumstances.

Atoms have what are known as electron shells, which are the levels that an electron is able to occupy.

Electrons cannot exist in between these shells; instead they jump from one to the next instantaneously. Each electron shell can hold a different number of atoms. When a shell fills up, additional electrons fill the outer shells. The outermost shell of any atom is called the valence shell, and it is the electrons in this shell that interact with the electrons of other atoms. The important thing about the valence shell is that each electron shell has a specific number of electrons that it can hold, and it wants to hold that many.

When atoms join, their connecting valence electrons take up two valence shell spots, one on each atom.

This means that the fewer electrons an atom has in its valence shell, the likelier it is to interact with other atoms. Conversely, the more electrons it has, the less likely it is to interact.

Electrons can also momentarily jump from one electron shell to the next if they are hit with a burst of energy from a photon.

When photons hit atoms, the energy is briefly absorbed by the electrons, and this momentarily knocks them into higher "orbits." The particular "orbit" the electron is knocked into depends on the type of atom, and when the electron gives up its higher energy level it re-emits a photon at a slightly different wavelength than the one it absorbed, providing a characteristic signal of that atom and showing exactly what "orbit" the electron was knocked into.

This is the phenomenon responsible for spectral lines in light and is the reason we can tell what elements make up stars and planets just by looking at them.

Unlike protons and neutrons, electrons are a fundamental particle all on their own. They are known as leptons.

Electrons have a negative charge that is generally balanced out by the positive charge of their atom's protons.

Charged atoms, which have either gained or lost an electron for various reasons, are called ions.

Ions, like isotopes, have the same properties that the regular element does; they simply have different tendencies towards reacting with other atoms. Electrons have a mass of 9.1094×10^{-31} kg and a $-\frac{1}{2}$ spin.

Element

The concept of chemical element is related to that of chemical substance. A chemical element is specifically a substance which is composed of a single type of atom.

A chemical element is characterized by a particular number of protons in the nuclei of its atoms. This number is known as the atomic number of the element. For example, all atoms with 6 protons in their nuclei are atoms of the chemical element carbon, and all atoms with 92 protons in their nuclei are atoms of the element uranium.

Compound

A compound is a substance with a particular ratio of atoms of particular chemical elements which determines its composition, and a particular organization which determines chemical properties.

For example, water is a compound containing hydrogen and oxygen in the ratio of two to one, with the oxygen atom between the two hydrogen atoms, and an angle of 104.5° between them. Compounds are formed and interconverted by chemical reactions.

Substance

A chemical substance is a kind of matter with a definite composition and set of properties.

Strictly speaking, a mixture of compounds, elements or compounds and elements is not a chemical substance, but it may be called a chemical. Most of the

SCIENCE

substances we encounter in our daily life are some kind of mixture; for example: air, alloys, biomass, etc.

Nomenclature of substances is a critical part of the language of chemistry. Generally it refers to a system for naming chemical compounds.

Earlier in the history of chemistry substances were given names by their discoverer, which often led to some confusion and difficulty. However, today the IUPAC system of chemical nomenclature allows chemists to specify by name specific compounds amongst the vast variety of possible chemicals.

The standard nomenclature of chemical substances is set by the International Union of Pure and Applied Chemistry (IUPAC). There are well-defined systems in place for naming chemical species. Organic compounds are named according to the organic nomenclature system. Inorganic compounds are named according to the inorganic nomenclature system. In addition the Chemical Abstracts Service has devised a method to index chemical substance. In this scheme each chemical substance is identifiable by a number known as CAS registry number.

Molecule

Molecules are two or more atoms join through a chemical bond to form chemicals.

Molecules differ from atoms in that molecules can be further broken down into smaller pieces and into elements while atoms cannot. (This was actually the 18th century definition of an atom: a recognizable structure that could no longer be broken down into smaller bits.)

Atoms are joined into molecules in two main ways: through covalent bonds and through ionic bonds.

Covalent bonds are the primary type of chemical bond that forms molecules. They occur when atoms with only partially filled valence electron shells, an atom's outermost electron shell, come together to share electrons. Hydrogen atoms, for instance, each have only one electron, while their valence shell is capable of holding two. When two hydrogen atoms come together each share the other's electron, using it to occupy its valence shell's free space forming the H2 molecule: hydrogen gas.

Not all covalent bond's are the same.

Different atoms have different levels of positive charge coming from in their nuclei, and although, under normal circumstances, the negative charge of the atom's electrons balances that out (keeping the atom electrically neutral) the chemical bonding process has a way of exploiting this situation. If we look at the H2 molecule again, everyday experience tells us that it has a strong tendency to seek out and bond with oxygen (O) molecules forming H2O, or water. There are two main reasons for this. The first comes from the regular old covalent bonds that are already holding H2 together. If bonded to another atom, hydrogen gains the ability to form a new valence shell that can hold six electrons. Since oxygen is the only molecule to naturally have six electrons in its valence shell, it is the most eager to bond with hydrogen. However, oxygen also has 8 protons in its nucleus compared to the total of 2 in the H2 molecule. This means that as the atoms come closer and prepare to bond, the electrons from both atoms are pulled closer to the oxygen molecule and farther from the hydrogen. An atom's proclivity to pull electrons towards itself is called its electronegativity, and this process creates polar covalent bonds. Due to this connection, polar covalent bonds are the strongest molecular bond, which is why molecules like water are so prevalent in our solar system and, likely, throughout the galaxy.

One very interesting aspect of polar covalent bonds is the hydrogen bond.

When a hydrogen atom bonds with another electronegative atom, the newly created molecule develops an intense polar attraction to all other electronegative atoms. This attraction works almost like a magnet with one end of the molecule exhibiting a positive charge (due to the effects of the polar covalent bonds pulling all the electrons towards one end of the molecule) and the other end exhibiting a negative charge. This phenomenon is responsible for, among other things, the way water molecules stick to each other so readily. This is why you can fill a glass of water to a millimeter or so above the rim before it spills.

Hydrogen bonds are also responsible for how hydrophilic and hydrophobic molecules react to being mixed with water.

Hydrophilic molecules are molecules like NaCl (salt) which exhibit their own strong charge for reasons we will discuss in a moment. The charged salt molecules mix eagerly with the charged water molecules due to the extra pull of the hydrogen bond. Conversely, hydrophobic molecules such as oil will not mix with water because they are neutrally charged and do not like charged molecules. This is the reason you have to shake up an oil based salad dressing each time you use it. Oil and the water never truly mix, and quickly separate.

A very different type of bond between atoms is called the ionic bond.

Ionic bonds only occur between ions, atoms that are either positively or negatively charged due to having an unequal number of protons and electrons. Ionic bonds always occur between metals and non-metals, such as the gas chlorine (Cl) and the alkaline metal sodium (Na). In their normal states, neither of these elements are ions, but when they approach, the sodium gives the chlorine one of its electrons forming Cl- and Na+ ions, which subsequently become attracted. Since no electrons are actually lost, the molecule still technically has a neutral charge; it is only the atoms that are charged.

In ionic bonds it is always the metal which gives its electron to the non-metal.

Additionally, in a diluted or liquid form, molecules that are created like this will always conduct electricity. This is why salt water can make such a good conductor.

Ions and salts

An ion is a charged species, an atom or a molecule, that has lost or gained one or more electrons.

Positively charged cations (e.g. sodium cation Na+) and negatively charged anions (e.g. chloride Cl−) can form a crystalline lattice of neutral salts (e.g. sodium chloride NaCl). Examples of polyatomic ions that do not split up during acid-base reactions are hydroxide (OH−) and phosphate (PO43−).

Ions in the gaseous phase are often known as plasma.

Acidity and basicity

A substance can often be classified as an acid or a base. There are several different theories which explain acid-base behavior. The simplest is Arrhenius theory.

The Arrhenius theory states than an acid is a substance that produces hydronium ions when it is dissolved in water, and a base is one that produces hydroxide ions when dissolved in water. According to Brønsted–Lowry acid-base theory, acids are substances that donate a positive hydrogen ion to another substance in a chemical reaction; by extension, a base is the substance which receives that hydrogen ion.

A third common theory is Lewis acid-base theory, which is based on the formation of new chemical bonds.

Lewis theory explains that an acid is a substance capable of accepting a pair of electrons from another substance during the process of bond formation, while a base is a substance which can provide a pair of electrons to form a new bond. According to concept as per Lewis, the crucial things being exchanged are charges. There are several other ways in which a substance may be classified as an acid or a base, as is evident in the history of this concept

Acid strength is commonly measured by two methods. The most common is pH.

One measurement, based on the Arrhenius definition of acidity, is pH, which is a measurement of the hydronium ion concentration in a solution, as expressed on a negative logarithmic scale. Thus, solutions that have a low pH have a high hydronium ion concentration, and can be said to be more acidic. The other measurement, based on the Brønsted–Lowry definition, is the acid dissociation constant (K_a), which measure the relative ability of a substance to act as an acid under the Brønsted–Lowry definition of an acid. That is, substances with a higher K_a are more likely to donate hydrogen ions in chemical reactions than those with lower K_a values.

Phase

In addition to the specific chemical properties that distinguish chemical classifications, chemicals can exist in several phases.

For the most part, the chemical classifications are independent of these bulk phase classifications; however, some more exotic phases are incompatible with certain chemical properties. A phase is a set of states of a chemical system that have similar bulk structural properties, over a range of conditions, such as pressure or temperature.

Physical properties, such as density and refractive index tend to fall within values characteristic of the phase. The phase of matter is defined by the phase transition, which is when energy put into, or taken out of the system goes into rearranging the structure of the system, instead of changing the bulk conditions.

Phase can be continuous.

Sometimes the distinction between phases can be continuous instead of having a discrete boundary, here the matter is considered to be in a supercritical state. When three states meet based on the conditions, it is known as a triple point and since this is invariant, it is a convenient way to define a set of conditions.

The most familiar examples of phases are solids, liquids, and gases. Many substances exhibit multiple solid phases. For example, there are three phases of solid iron (alpha, gamma, and delta) that vary based on temperature and pressure. A principle difference between solid phases is the crystal structure, or arrangement, of the atoms. Another phase commonly encountered in the study of chemistry is the aqueous phase, which is the state of substances dissolved in aqueous solution (that is, in water).

Less familiar phases include plasmas, Bose-Einstein condensates and fermionic condensates and the paramagnetic and ferromagnetic phases of magnetic materials. While most familiar phases deal with three-dimensional systems, it is also possible to define analogs in two-dimensional systems, which has received attention for its relevance to systems in biology.

Redox

Redox is a concept related to the ability of atoms of various substances to lose or gain electrons.

Substances that can oxidize other substances are said to be oxidative and are known as oxidizing agents, oxidants or oxidizers. An oxidant removes electrons from another substance. Similarly, substances that can reduce other substances are said to be reductive and are known as reducing agents, reductants, or reducers.

A reductant transfers electrons to another substance, and is thus oxidized itself. And because it "donates" electrons it is also called an electron donor.

> Oxidation and reduction properly refer to a change in oxidation number—the actual transfer of electrons may never occur. Thus, oxidation is better defined as an increase in oxidation number, and reduction as a decrease in oxidation number.

Bonding

Electron atomic and molecular orbitals

Atoms sticking together in molecules or crystals are said to be bonded with one another.

> A chemical bond may be visualized as the multipole balance between the positive charges in the nuclei and the negative charges oscillating about them. More than simple attraction and repulsion, the energies and distributions characterize the availability of an electron to bond to another atom.

A chemical bond can be a covalent bond, an ionic bond, a hydrogen bond or just because of Van der Waals force.

> Each of these kinds of bond is ascribed to some potential. These potentials create the interactions which hold atoms together in molecules or crystals. In many simple compounds, Valence Bond Theory, the Valence Shell Electron Pair Repulsion model (VSEPR), and the concept of oxidation number can explain molecular structure and composition.

Reaction

During chemical reactions, bonds between atoms break and form, resulting in different substances with different properties.

> In a blast furnace, iron oxide, a compound, reacts with carbon monoxide to form iron, a chemical elements, and carbon dioxide.

> When a chemical substance is transformed as a result of its interaction with another or energy, a chemical reaction is said to have occurred. Chemical reaction is therefore a concept related to the 'reaction' of a substance when it comes in close contact, as a mixture or a solution; exposure to some form of energy, or, both. It results in some energy exchange between the constituents of the reaction as well with the system environment which may be designed vessels which are often laboratory glassware.

Chemical reactions can result in the formation or dissociation of molecules, that is, molecules breaking apart to form two or more smaller molecules, or rearrangement of atoms within or across molecules.

> Chemical reactions usually involve the making or breaking of chemical bonds. Oxidation, reduction, dissociation, acid-base neutralization and molecular rear-

rangement are some of the commonly used kinds of chemical reactions.

A chemical reaction can be symbolically depicted through a chemical equation. While in a non-nuclear chemical reaction the number and kind of atoms on both sides of the equation are equal, for a nuclear reaction, this holds true only for the nuclear particles viz. protons and neutrons.

The sequence of steps in which the reorganization of chemical bonds may be taking place in the course of a chemical reaction is called its mechanism.

A chemical reaction can be envisioned to take place in several steps, each of which may have a different speed. Many reaction intermediates with variable stability can thus be envisaged during a reaction. Reaction mechanisms are proposed to explain the kinetics and the relative product mix of a reaction. Many physical chemists specialize in exploring and proposing the mechanisms of various chemical reactions. Several empirical rules, like the Woodward-Hoffmann rules often come handy while proposing a mechanism for a chemical reaction.

Equilibrium

Although the concept of equilibrium is widely used across sciences, in the context of chemistry, it arises whenever a number of different states of the chemical composition are possible.

For example, in a mixture of several chemical compounds that can react, or, when a substance can be present in more than one kind of phase.

A system of chemical substances at equilibrium even though having an unchanging composition is most often not static; molecules of the substances continue to react, thus creating a dynamic equilibrium. Thus the concept describes the state in which the parameters such as chemical composition remain unchanged over time. Chemicals present in biological systems are invariably not at equilibrium; but are far from equilibrium.

Science

The Periodic Table

The periodic table contains the known chemical elements displayed in a special tabular arrangement based on their electron configurations, atomic numbers and recurring chemical properties.

The first semblance of a periodic table was by Antoine Lavoisier in 1789. He published a list or table of the 33 chemical elements known as of that time. He grouped the elements into earths, non-metals, gases and metals. Several chemists in the next century looked for a better classification method resulting in the periodic table as we have it today.

Structure of the Periodic Table

The standard periodic table as it is today is an 18 column by 7 rows table containing the main chemical elements. Beneath that is a smaller 15 column by 2 rows table. The periodic table can be broken down into 4 rectangular blocks: the P block is by the right, S block is left, D block is at the middle and the F block is underneath that. The elements in the blocks are based on which sub-shell the last electron resides.

The chemical elements on the table are arranged in order of increasing atomic number, which refers to the number of protons of the element. The periodic table can be used to study the chemical behavior of chemical elements, which makes it a very important tool widely used in chemistry.

The periodic table contains only chemical elements. Mixtures, compounds or small atomic particles of elements are not included. Each element on the table has a unique atomic number, which represents the number of protons contained in the element's nucleus.

A new period or row begins when an element has a new electron shell with a first electron. Columns or groups are based on the configuration of electrons of the atom. Elements that have an equal number of atoms in a specific sub-shell are listed under the same column. For example, selenium and oxygen both have 4 electrons in their outermost sub shell and so are listed under the P column. Elements with similar properties are listed in the same group although some elements in the same period can also share similar properties too. Since the elements grouped together have related properties, one can easily predict the property of an element if the properties of the surrounding elements are already known.

Rows are Periods

The rows of the periodic table are called periods. Elements on a row have the same number of electron shells or atomic orbitals. Elements on the first row have just one atomic orbital, elements on the second row have 2, and so it goes until the elements on the seventh row that have 7 electron shells or atomic orbitals.

Columns are Groups

Columns from up to down in the table are called groups. The columns in the D, P and S blocks are called groups. Elements within a group have equal number of electrons in their outermost electron shell or orbital. The electrons on the outer shell are called valence electrons and there are the electrons that combine with other elements in a chemical reaction.

The Periodic table contains natural and synthesized elements

The elements up to californium are natural existing elements (94) while the rest were laboratory synthesized. Chemists are still working to produce elements beyond the present 118th element, ununoctium. 114 of the 118 elements on the table have been officially recognized by the International Union of Pure and Applied Chemistry (IUPAC). Elements listed on the table under 113, 115, 117 and 118 have been synthesized but are yet to officially recognized by the IUPAC and are only known by their systematic element names.

Group → ↓ Period	1	2	3	4	5	6	7	8	9	10	11	12	13	14	15	16	17	18
1	1 H																	2 He
2	3 Li	4 Be											5 B	6 C	7 N	8 O	9 F	10 Ne
3	11 Na	12 Mg											13 Al	14 Si	15 P	16 S	17 Cl	18 Ar
4	19 K	20 Ca	21 Sc	22 Ti	23 V	24 Cr	25 Mn	26 Fe	27 Co	28 Ni	29 Cu	30 Zn	31 Ga	32 Ge	33 As	34 Se	35 Br	36 Kr
5	37 Rb	38 Sr	39 Y	40 Zr	41 Nb	42 Mo	43 Tc	44 Ru	45 Rh	46 Pd	47 Ag	48 Cd	49 In	50 Sn	51 Sb	52 Te	53 I	54 Xe
6	55 Cs	56 Ba		72 Hf	73 Ta	74 W	75 Re	76 Os	77 Ir	78 Pt	79 Au	80 Hg	81 Tl	82 Pb	83 Bi	84 Po	85 At	86 Rn
7	87 Fr	88 Ra		104 Rf	105 Db	106 Sg	107 Bh	108 Hs	109 Mt	110 Ds	111 Rg	112 Cn	113 Uut	114 Fl	115 Uup	116 Lv	117 Uus	118 Uuo

Lanthanides	57 La	58 Ce	59 Pr	60 Nd	61 Pm	62 Sm	63 Eu	64 Gd	65 Tb	66 Dy	67 Ho	68 Er	69 Tm	70 Yb	71 Lu
Actinides	89 Ac	90 Th	91 Pa	92 U	93 Np	94 Pu	95 Am	96 Cm	97 Bk	98 Cf	99 Es	100 Fm	101 Md	102 No	103 Lr

Science

Chemistry and Energy

In the context of chemistry, energy is an attribute of a substance as a consequence of its atomic, molecular or aggregate structure. Since a chemical transformation is accompanied by a change in one or more of these kinds of structure, it is invariably accompanied by an increase or decrease of energy of the substances involved.

> Some energy is transferred between the surroundings and the reactants of the reaction as heat or light; thus the products of a reaction may have more or less energy than the reactants.

Exergonic, Endergonic, Exothermic and Endothermic

> A reaction is said to be exergonic if the final state is lower on the energy scale than the initial state; for endergonic reactions the situation is the reverse. A reaction is said to be exothermic if the reaction releases heat to the surroundings; for endothermic reactions, the reaction absorbs heat from the surroundings.

Chemical reactions are invariably not possible unless the reactants surmount an energy barrier known as the activation energy.

> The speed of a chemical reaction (at given temperature T) is related to the activation energy E, by the Boltzmann's population factor $e - E/kT$ - that is the probability of molecule to have energy greater than than, or equal to E at the given temperature T. This exponential dependence of a reaction rate on temperature is known as the Arrhenius equation. The activation energy necessary for a chemical reaction can be in the form of heat, light, electricity or mechanical force as ultrasound.

Ecology

Ecology is the scientific study of the relationship between the Earth and its life forms. The purpose of ecology is to understand the structures that occur in nature.

> Ecologists study the planet's ecosystems, the various communities of living things (biotic) and non-living structures (abiotic) that occur in localized areas throughout the world. The purpose of ecology is to understand the organizational structures that occur spontaneously in nature. Within an ecosystem there are different levels of organization which are broken down by relative size. Each ecosystem is composed of communities of animals, and within each community exist numerous populations, or individual species groups.

Ecosystems Ecology

Ecosystems ecology studies areas that can be differentiated from neighboring areas by the types of rocks, soil and other non-living features, as well as the types of plants and animals adapted to live there.

A desert ecosystem may boarder an arid grassland ecosystem, which in turn may boarder a forest ecosystem. The purpose of ecosystems ecology is to analyze the system of interactions the animals and plants in a particular area have with the non-living portions environment. It also focuses heavily on local evolution, studying what traits are favored within particular ecosystems and why.

Ecosystems can be qualified.

Many quantifiable factors go into making an ecosystem. Abiotic components are things such average sunlight, temperature, average rainfall and moisture levels, soil composition and other similar factors. Similarly, biotic components consist of the number and type of primary producers (generally plants), secondary producers (herbivores) and tertiary producers (carnivores and omnivores). All this information can be quantified. For example, ecologists can calculate the amount of energy in a system by studying the average quantity of sunlight, the efficiency of photosynthesis in local plants, calories that exist in prey animals, nutrients absorbed by bacteria from breaking down dead predators and so on. Provided all the factors have been accounted for, this type of quantitative analysis of ecosystems can help ecologists determine factors such as the efficiency of the food web and the maximum supportable population. It can also help determine accurate ways to repair damaged ecosystems.

Community Ecology

Community ecology looks at similar regions to ecosystems ecology but focuses primarily on the biotic factors, ignoring the abiotic.
In ecological terms a community describes the interactions of several species in a local area. Ecologists define these interactions between species in several ways: mutualism, interaction where species benefit such as between bees and flowering plants; commensalism, interaction where one species benefits and the other neither notices nor minds; competition, interaction where species are harmed; and predation or parasitism, interaction where one species is benefitted while the other is harmed such as predators attacking prey or herbivores eating plants.

A local food web, is a graphical representation showing who eats what in nature.

To ecologists, however, food webs are much more specific, showing the transfer of energy from organism to organism. Energy moves from lower trophic levels to higher ones. Trophic levels are the various positions that plants and animals occupy within the food web relative to other plants and animals that they want to eat or that want to eat them. Plants, for instance, would have a lower trophic level than grazing animals such as deer. Similarly, deer would have lower trophic levels than wolves.

Within communities species can be affected by changes either directly (such as when their main predator ate them) or indirectly (such as their main predator has its numbers diminished by a new and even bigger predator). There are also cascading effects on communities, such as, when a dominant herbivorous species dies out and all its former prey (both plant and animal) increase drastically in number.

Each organism occupies a trophic level (or position) in the food chain.

A food chain represents a succession of organisms that eat another organism and are, in turn, eaten themselves. The number of steps an organism is from the start of the chain is a measure of its trophic level. The simplest is the first trophic level (level 1) is plants, then herbivores (level 2), and then carnivores (level 3).

A trophic pyramid (a) and a simplified community food web (b) illustrating ecological relations among creatures that are typical of a northern Boreal terrestrial ecosystem. The trophic pyramid roughly represents the biomass (usually measured as total dry-weight) at each level. Plants generally have the greatest biomass. Names of trophic categories are shown to the right of the pyramid. Some ecosystems, such as many wetlands, do not organize as a strict pyramid, because aquatic plants are not as productive as long-lived terrestrial plants such as trees. Ecological trophic pyramids are typically one of three kinds: 1) pyramid of numbers, 2) pyramid of biomass, or 3) pyramid of energy

Population Ecology

Population Ecology studies a single species and the primary factor is population size.

Getting even more specific is population ecology, which focuses on only one species either within a community or across a large space. The primary characteristic of a population is its size. Population sizes can change due to an imbalance in the number of births and deaths as well as plants and animals emigrating to new areas.

Ecologists who study populations will generally model their growth rates to make predictions about the species. One method is the exponential growth model, which looks at current population trends and, assuming they will remain constant, shows the increase or decrease in population over numerous generations. The other method is the logistic growth model, which slows reproduction when populations reach a certain density and increases it when they drop below a certain density to account for the increase in predators and decrease in the food supply that often follows massive population growth.

Natural Selection and Adaptation

Natural selection and adaptation are one of the fundamental teachings of evolution. Natural selection is the non-random gradual process that biological traits become more common or less common among a population.

The theory of natural selection was made popular by Charles Darwin and was first introduced in his 1859 book; The Origin of Species.

As species and organisms evolve, some mutations and changes in the genomes occur as they interact with their environments. These changes and mutations can be passed from the organism to its offspring. In time, individual organisms or living beings with particular traits or genome variants may survive and produce offspring more successfully than individuals with different traits or genome variants. As this process goes on, the population slowly evolves as individuals with weak traits relative to their environment die out or are replaced by individuals with the right traits or mutations to survive. This is why the process of natural selection is also sometimes called the survival of fittest.

Over time as species and organisms continue to react to their environment and develop traits and genome variants to suit their environment they may become specialized to suit a particular environment niche, and new species may even be produced. Natural selection is thus an important pillar of evolution although it is not the only process that lead to evolution.

Natural selection differs with artificial selection because the latter involves the purposeful selection of specific favorable traits by humans.

With natural selection, the individual organism doesn't make the choice, but the changing environment determines which traits are necessary for survival and individual organisms that lack the required traits would die out.

Not all variants and mutations affect the survival of the individual.

For example, the difference in eye color among a population such as among humans is not necessarily a survival factor. However, a rabbit that develops the trait of running faster and passes it onto its offspring, has improved chances of escape and survival from predators than rabbits that do not. The same would be true for algae that successfully develop the trait or ability to extract more energy from sunlight, such algae would outgrow others without this trait.

Adaptation

Adaptation is a process in which an organism evolves to be better able to live and survive in its habitat or environments.

Adaptation is closely related to natural selection and it covers both the state of being adapted to the environment and the process that led to the adaptation. Adaptation is also a fundamental teaching of evolution as popularized by

Charles Darwin.

Organisms existing in their various environments face several challenges that they must adapt to survive. An organism must develop observable phenotype traits in response to the conditions imposed on it by its environment for it to survive and thrive.

The ability of an organism to adapt is thus closely linked to its fitness and survival. Adaptation is not exactly simple or fast. It may take a period of small steps for the entire process to be complete and for the organism to be fully adapted. During all the stages of adaptation and evolution, the organism has to be viable to be able to survive the process.

Adaptation is a process in which the phenotype of the organism changes to better suit the environment. There are many classical examples of adaptation. An animal that develops thick fur to survive the cold environment has adapted, just as the case of an animal that develops effective camouflage techniques to hide itself from predators.

Adaptation can be behavioral, structural or physiological.

Structural adaptation has to do with changes in physical features such as body covering, physical defense mechanism, size and shape and some internal restructuring.

Physiological adaptations allow the organism to do perform unique functions such as secreting slime, making venom or phototropism. Physiological adaptations include general functions such as temperature regulation, development and growth and ionic balance.

Behavioral adaptations include inherited behaviors and mannerisms as well as the ability to learn. Inherited behaviors are termed instinct and may include mating style, food search and vocalizations.

Basic Physics

Kinetic and Mechanical Energy

The kinetic energy of an object is the energy it possesses due to its motion.

Kinetic energy is the work needed to accelerate a body of a given mass from rest to a stated velocity. Like all forms of energy, kinetic energy is measured in joules. Kinetic energy can be imparted to an object when an energy source is tapped to accelerate it. It can also happen when one object with kinetic energy slams into another object and kinetic energy from the first object is transferred to the second.

However it happens, imparting kinetic energy to an object causes it to accelerate. In this way movement is nothing more than an indication of the amount of kinetic energy an object has. An object will hold onto its kinetic energy until it is able to transfer it to something else, which allows it to slow down again.

As long as an object has the same level of kinetic energy, it will move at a consistent velocity forever. This is Newton's first law of motion.

The transfer of kinetic energy from one object to another can occur in many ways.

The transfer of kinetic energy can be as simple and mundane as a baseball flying through the air—interacting with all the various molecules of oxygen, carbon dioxide, nitrogen and all the other gasses that make up our atmosphere, and transferring its kinetic energy to them—speeding them up and slowing itself down in the process. Or it can be as chaotic as a speeding truck losing control on an icy road and slamming into a wall.

Different types of interactions between objects appear to be different but are in fact the same.

The interaction between the baseball and the air and between the truck and the wall are only superficially different. One appears more chaotic than the other only because of the differences in mass between a baseball and a truck and the differences in "negative energy" possessed by free-floating air molecules compared to a solid wall. At its most basic, however, the same events are taking place in both examples. Molecules both in the wall and the air scatter when the kinetic energy they receive causes them to move, and this causes both heat and sound to be produced.

Kinetic energy can be calculated with the formula $KE = \frac{1}{2}mv^2$ where m is the mass of the object in kilograms, and v is its velocity in meters/second.

Kinetic energy increases by the square of an objects velocity.

One important aspect of kinetic energy that makes it so potentially destructive is that the kinetic energy relative to not increase on pace with its velocity, but rather, relative to the square of its velocity. If you double an object's velocity, you will quadruple the kinetic energy it possesses ($2^2=4$). If you quadruple the velocity, you increase the kinetic energy by sixteen times ($4^2=16$). This leads to relatively small masses possessing very high kinetic energy levels when they are accelerated to only nominally high speeds. This is one reason why modern kinetic energy weapons (such as firearms) are able to cause large amounts of damage while being extremely compact.

Mechanical Energy

Mechanical energy is the ability of an object to do work.

When discussing energy it is important to take a moment to understand mechanical energy and how it relates to the objects it interacts with. Mechanical energy is not a separate type of energy in the way that potential energy and kinetic energy differ.

Mechanical energy is the potential energy available to an object added to all of the kinetic energy available to it, providing a total energy output.

For instance, in our description of potential energy there is the example of a pole-vaulter hanging in mid-air with her pole bent at a near right angle to the ground. The bend in the pole-vaulter's pole contains elastic potential energy, which will help her clear the bar. However, that is not the only source of energy the pole-vaulter is restricted to. For anyone who has ever seen a track and field competition, you know that pole-vaulters take long, running starts before planting their poles in the ground. This imparts kinetic energy to the runners body, and it is that kinetic energy plus the pole's elastic potential energy that are added together in mid-air to impart the total mechanical energy that drives the pole-vaulter high into the air and over the bar.

Potential Energy

There are two main types of potential energy: gravitational potential energy and elastic potential energy.

Potential energy is the potential an object has to act on other objects. As gravitational potential energy, the object is raised off the ground and is waiting for the force of gravity pulling at $9.8 m/s^2$, to grab hold of it and pull it towards the Earth.

This type of energy is very common in everyday life. It describes everything from a book falling off its shelf to a child tripping on a crack in the sidewalk. Because gravitational potential energy is so common, the equation describing it PEgrav = mass * g * height should not be hard to figure out since it contains only easily observable features of matter: an object's mass, the force of gravity (g), and the object's height off the ground when it started falling.
Note that the height does not have to be measured from the ground. Any point can be chosen—such as a table top or even a point in mid-air—if you are only concerned with the energy an object would have if it fell from the point it was currently at to the point you have chosen.

Gravitational Potential Energy Example

If we take the example of a 1kg weight positioned at a height of 1 meter above the surface of Earth (where the gravity is $9.8 m/s^2$—try this on Mars and you will get a different result), we end with the equation PEgrav = 1 * 9.8 * 1, which equals 9.8 joules of gravitational potential energy. A 1g weight positioned at the same height would be PEgrav = .001 * 9.8 * 1 or .0098J of potential energy, while a 1kg weight positioned a kilometer up would equal PEgrav = 1 * 9.8 * 1000 or 9800J of potential energy.

From this equation you may have picked up on the fact that the height an object is raised, is directly proportional to the amount of gravitational potential energy it has. Take a 1kg object and raise it to 5m, and you get 49J of potential energy. Double that to 10m, and you get 98J. Triple it to 15m and you will get 147J—three times the original 49J.

Elastic Potential Energy

Elastic potential energy occurs when an object is stretched or compressed out of its normal "resting" shape. The quantity of energy that will be released when it finally returns to rest is the quantity of elastic potential energy it has while stretched or compressed.

A common example of elastic potential energy is when an archer draws back the string of his bow. The farther back the bowstring is pulled, the more it will stretch. The more it stretches the more potential energy it will have waiting to send into the arrow.

Elastic potential energy of an object can be determined using Hooke's law of elasticity. Hooke's law states that F = -kx where F is the force the material will exert as it returns to its resting state measured in Newtons, x is amount of displacement the material undergoes measured in meters, and k is the spring constant and is measured in Newtons/meter.

To determine the potential energy of an elastic or springy material you use the equation PE = 1/2 kx^2. According to this equation, an object such as a spring with a spring constant of 5N/m that is stretched 3 meters past its resting point would have a potential energy of 22.5J. That is, ½ * 5 * 3^2 = 2.5 * 9 = 22.5J. Remember that elastic potential energy affects much more than just what you would consider elastic or springy material such as rubber bands, bungee cords and springs. There is elastic potential energy in a pole-vaulter's pole at the point where she is in the air and hanging onto a pole that is bent nearly sideways. In the next instant, her forward momentum will be boosted by the conversion of her pole's potential energy into kinetic energy, pushing her over the bar. Similarly, when a hockey player shoots the puck, he drags his stick along the ice as it moves forward, bending the shaft backwards slightly. This adds extra force to the puck as the stick snaps forward back into its normal resting position.

Human Body Science

Energy: Work and Power

In the simplest terms, energy is the ability to do work.

Energy allows objects and people to effect the physical world and displace (or move) other objects or people.

Work in the physics sense is a very specific concept.

It is measured in joules, which are defined as being 1 Newton of force that displaces something by 1 meter. (J = Nm) As the mass of the object being displaced varies, the quantity of work in joules required to move it a meter will vary too.

To determine the quantity of work being done, you can use the equation $W = F * d * \cos\Theta$.

This defines work as the force applied, multiplied by the distance the object was displaced, multiplied by the cosine of Θ (Theta).

The force is measured in Newtons. Distance is measured in meters. The tricky part of this equation is determining the cosine of Θ. Θ represents the difference in angle between the vector (or direction) the force is acting in and the vector the displacement is occurring. That means that there are really only three possible values for Θ.

If the force is pushing or pulling in one direction, and the object being displaced is moving in that same direction, then there is no difference in angle between the vectors and $\Theta=0°$. This is the sort of force you get when a child pulls her sled across a snowy field. The direction the child is pulling and the direction the sled is traveling are the same. Since $\cos 0 = 1$ the quantity of work is determined simply by multiplying the force and the displacement.

Note that the angle of the vectors is determined by their relationship, and not to an ideal flat surface. That is, if the child is pulling her sled up a steep hill rather than across a field, the angle of Θ is still going to be 0° since the force she exerts on the sled and the sled itself are still traveling in the same direction.

The second possibility is when the force vector acts in the opposite direction of the object's displacement. This gives what is called "negative work" because the energy is working to hinder the object from moving rather than to help it. In this instance $\Theta=180°$ since the vector in which the force is acting and the vector in which the object is moving are opposite. This force is most commonly observed when dealing with friction. It is the reason that hockey pucks and soccer balls will not travel forever; the force of friction exerted by the ice and by the grass is acting in the opposite direction.

The final difference in vectors is when the force being exerted on an object is at a right angle to its displacement. Here, $\Theta=90°$. You can picture this as a waitress carrying a tray of drinks over to your table, and it provides for some odd conclusions. Since the force we are talking about is the force the waitress is using to hold the tray vertically, but the displacement vector of the tray is horizontally across the room, we find that the force the waitress exerts no work at all. It is not responsible for moving the tray horizontally towards your table.

This is represented mathematically with the fact that the cos90 = 0, meaning that the original equation W = F * d * cosΘ would be W = F * d * 0. Without adding any additional information, it is obvious that work is going to equal zero joules.

A different way to imagine this is to think of cargo in the back of a truck.

It took work to load the cargo up onto the truck from the ground (the force vector and the displacement vector were both pointing in the same direction), but once the cargo was loaded, no additional work was required to keep it there. The truck could drive from one end of the country to the other, but zero joules of work would be exerted keeping the cargo in place in the back of the truck.

When you add a unit of time to your calculations of work, you get a new classification: power.

Power is the rate at which work is done. The equation that measures power, is power = work/time. In this equation work is measured in joules, time is measured in seconds and power is measured in watts.
Since, as we noted above, one joule is the same as one Newton multiplied by one meter, this equation can also be written as power=(force*displacement)/time where force is measured in Newtons and displacement is measured in meters. However, this opens further possibilities. Since the math does not care if we first multiply force with displacement before dividing the whole thing by time, or we divide displacement by time, and then multiply the answer by force, we find the equation can also be written as power = force(displacement/time).

Given that displacement is measured in meters and the time in seconds, what we are really saying here is that power equals the amount of force applied to an object multiplied by that object's velocity (m/s).

Thus we get two equations describing power: power = work/time and power=force*velocity.

By definition, power has an inverse relationship with time; the less time that it takes for the work to be done, the more power is being applied. Power also has a direct relationship with force and velocity. Increase either the quantity of force being applied to an object, or the speed at which it is traveling, and you have increased the power.

Defining Force and Newton's Three Laws

In physics force is the term given to anything that has the power to act on an object, causing its displacement in one direction or another.

> to identify accurately, and therefore it took thousands of years to identify accurately and describe them. It was not until the 17th century that Isaac Newton described the basic physical forces and show how they acted on matter.
>
> Force is measured using the unit Newton (N). One Newton can be defined with the formula $1N = 1kg(1m/s^2)$. In other words, if you accelerate a kilogram of matter by one meter per second per second, you have exerted one Newton of force on it.

Newton developed three laws to explain the interactions of matter he observed. The first is often known as the "Law of Inertia."

> It states that an object at rest will stay at rest, and an object in motion will stay in motion, unless a force acts on it to change its state. This means that if you fire a spaceship out into the vacuum of space, and keep it clear from planets and stars that will apply force to it, the ship will keep going at the same speed forever.
>
> This tendency to stay moving or stay at rest is known as inertia. Inertia is directly related to an object's mass; the more mass an object has, the more inertia it will have and the harder it will be to speed it up or slow it down. This is implied by the equation defining one Newton of force, but it is also obvious in everyday life. You have to exert more force to push a box of books across the floor than you would to push a box of clothes the same size. The box of books has more mass, so it has more inertia. Similarly, a baseball player can easily catch and stop a baseball thrown at over 100km/hr. If you were to ask that same player to stop a truck traveling at 100km/hr, you would get much less pleasant results.

One important thing to remember about force is that it is a vector quantity, meaning that it points in a specific direction.

> Set a one kilogram object down on a table and you will have the force of gravity pulling it down at one Newton, and the force of all the atoms in the table pushing it up at one Newton. This is said to be a state of equilibrium, and it causes no change to the object's velocity. However, if the table had been poorly built and was only capable of pushing up at .75 Newtons, the object would pull through, snapping the table at its weakest points, and fall until it found something that was capable of applying the needed force to hold it up against gravity.
>
> As such, an object can only be at rest if it has no forces acting on it, or if it has equal and opposite forces acting on it keeping it at equilibrium. If an unopposed force acts on an object, it will move.

Newton's second law deals with what happens when you have the sort of unbalanced forces that we just described.

It explains the movement of objects through the equation F=ma, where F is the force in Newtons, m is the object's mass in kilograms, and a is the object's acceleration in meters per second per second (m/s2).
Just like with Newton's first law, this equation shows that mass is a huge player when it comes to using a force to move objects. The larger the mass, the more force you will need to accelerate or decelerate it to the same velocity.

Newton's third law states simply that for every action there is an equal and opposite reaction.

This means that if I pound my hand down on my desk right now, my desk will also be hitting up at my hand with the exact same force. This may sound strange, but it is the reason that pounding your hand on your desk can damage your desk and hurt your hand at the same time. It is also the reason that baseball bats can snap while imparting force onto the ball, and why a moving car hitting stationary wall will damage both.

Force: Friction

Friction is the force that resists the motion of objects in relation to other objects.

When two surfaces move relative to each other, the force of friction is what slows them down. Friction applies to all matter, whether it is a book sliding down a slanting shelf, a soccer ball rolling on the ground or a baseball flying though the air. Friction is a constant opposing force that keeps things from traveling forever.

Several laws describe how friction works.

Amontons' first law of friction says that, "The force of friction is directly proportional to the applied load." His second law of friction says that, "The force of friction is independent of the apparent area of contact." Similarly, Coulomb's law of friction states that, "Kinetic friction is independent of the sliding velocity."

The two main types of Friction are static friction and kinetic friction.

Static friction is what you get when one stationary object is stacked on top of another stationary object, such as a book resting on a table. The static friction between the book and the table determines how much sticking power there is between them, and at what angle you would have to tilt the table before the force of gravity overpowers the force of friction and starts the book sliding.

To calculate the maximum amount of static friction possible before the book starts sliding, you use the formula $f_s = \mu_s F_n$ where f_s is the total amount of static friction, μ_s (pronounced "mu") is the coefficient of static friction and F_n is

Human Body Science

the "normal force," the force being exerted perpendicularly through the surface into the object resting on it, keeping the object from breaking through the surface.

Another way to examine static friction is to calculate the angle the table will have to reach before the book will start sliding.

This is also known as the angle of repose, and it can be calculated using the formula $\tan\theta = \muس$ where θ (pronounced "theta") is the angle of repose, and $\mu س$ is the coefficient of static friction.

Aside from determining the angles that books will slide off tables, calculating static friction allows tire manufacturers to determine how "grippy" their treads are. If there were no friction, the wheel would not be a functional tool because it would not push itself against the road while moving. The higher the coefficient of friction between the tire and the road, the more grip the tire has.

Kinetic friction is sort of the inverse of static friction.

It is the force that causes moving objects to slow down. Kinetic friction applies to two surfaces moving relative to one another such as the bottom of a snowboard and the snowy ground. It can be calculated using the same basic formula used to calculate static friction: $fk = \mu k Fn$ with the only differences being the sub-k marks replacing the sub-s marks of the previous equation, signifying kinetic friction.

As kinetic friction slows an object, the object's kinetic energy is transformed into heat.

Fundamental Forces: Electromagnetism

Electromagnetism is one of the four fundamental forces. It is far more common than gravity, but only if you know where to look.

Electromagnetism is responsible for nearly all interactions in which gravity plays no part. It is what holds negatively charged electrons in orbit around the positively charged protons in the nucleus of an atom. It is also the force that joins atoms to each other to create molecules.

It is also electromagnetism that is responsible for the fact that matter—which is made up of atoms and at the subatomic level is mostly empty space—feels solid.

When you sit down in your chair, it is the electromagnetic attraction between the chair's atoms and between your body's atoms that keep you from falling through the chair and, conversely, that keep the chair from passing through you.

Electromagnetic force acts through a field.

This type of field can occur as a result of positively or negatively charged atoms (ions), atoms which have either more or fewer electrons than protons causing their overall charge to be unbalanced. Magnetic fields can also be created by applying electric current to conductive material (such as wire) with a conductive core (such as a nail).

Electric current is nothing more than a steady flow of electrons, and by turning on the current you send electrons through the core.

This aligns all the atoms in the metal so that they are parallel, and this creates a magnetic field. When you turn the electric current off, the electrons stop flowing, and the atoms, no longer forced by the current to line up, cease to be magnetic.

All electromagnetic fields have a positive and a negative pole.

Even the Earth's magnetic field, which is caused by the convective forces in the planet's core, sends electrons out of its negative pole (in the geographic North Pole) and reaccepts them at its positive pole (in the geographic South Pole in Antarctica). The Earth's magnetic field, like all magnetic fields, is able to effect charged particles.

Magnetic fields move in one direction around a magnet.

This direction is always the same in relation to the flow of current from the negative to the positive poles, and it is easy to test the direction of the field using the "right hand rule." Close your fist and make a "thumbs up" sign with your right hand. The positive pole is represented by the tip of your thumb, the negative by the other end of your hand, and the direction of the magnetic field by where your closed fingers are. Thus, if you point your thumb at yourself, your magnet has current coming out its negative pole pointed towards you and looping back around to the positive pole pointed away from you, and the field is pointed counter-clockwise, which here is to your left.

The effects of a magnetic field do not go on forever but follow the inverse square law.

The farther you move from a magnetic field, the less its force will effect you. By moving x times away from a magnetic field, you feel $1/x2$ times less magnetism.

Closely related to the electromagnetic field is electromagnetic radiation.

This radiation can take many forms, the most familiar are light, radio waves that carry radio and broadcast television, microwaves that cook our food, x-rays that can image the insides or our bodies, and gamma rays that come down from space and would have killed us all long ago if it were not for the Earth's magnetic field interacting with them.

Electromagnetic radiation is created, according to James Clerk Maxwell, by the oscillations of electromagnetic fields, which create electromagnetic waves.

The wave's frequency (or how energetic it is) determines what part of the electromagnetic spectrum it occupies—whether it is a gamma ray, a blue light or a radio signal. Electromagnetic radiation is the same thing as light, with what we are used to as visible light being a range of specific frequencies within the electromagnetic spectrum, so all electromagnetic radiation moves at the speed of light.

At the quantum level, the electromagnetic force has a transfer particle moving between charged atoms, attracting and repelling them. The electromagnetic transfer particle is the photon.

Fundamental Forces: Gravity

Gravity may be the most commonly, consciously experienced force.

We can see its effects everyday when books fall off shelves, when stray baseballs arc downwards and crash through windows and when Australians time and again fail to fall off the bottom of the world and out into space. Gravity is also largely responsible for the structure of the universe. Without it, stars would not ignite and begin fusion reactions, planets would not condense out of dust and metal and most matter would have no attraction to other matter in any way. Without gravity, life would not exist.

It may seem strange to learn that gravity is the weakest of all forces given that it holds the entire galaxy together.

Still, even with the gravitational mass of the entire planet pulling on an object such as a ball—causing it to sit motionless on the floor rather than float aimlessly off into space—a toddler could easily pick it up and run off with it, and there would be nothing the planet could do about it. Match that with the force an electromagnet exerts on metal; there is no comparison.

The idea of gravity as a force was first formulated by Isaac Newton in the late 17th century.

Newton's ideas were further elaborated on in the early 20th century by Albert Einstein, who described gravity as the effect of mass warping the fabric of space-time. This process is often portrayed as a large ball creating a divot in a flat sheet of space-time. The divot curves space-time and can catch objects that would otherwise be traveling in straight lines and redirect or even capture them.

On Earth gravity pulls objects towards the center of the planet at 9.8 m/s².

The squared rate of time shows that gravity is by its nature a force causing acceleration. Every second, the force of gravity increases the speed of an object by an additional 9.8 m/s, provided nothing able to resist the force gets in its way.

In Einstein's view of the universe, gravity moved in waves, which traveled through space at the speed of light.

As a result, he demonstrated that the force of gravity would take time to reach the object it was acting on. If, for instance, the sun were to vanish suddenly from the solar system, it would take eight minutes for the Earth to go flying off into space—the same amount of time it would take for us to stop seeing the sun's light.

Another way to view gravity is through a series of transfer particles that interact with matter and draw it closer together.

Transfer particles come into play in quantum mechanics, and they replace gravity waves as the method of spreading the force through the universe. (Actually, replace is not the right word, as quantum mechanics shows that particles and waves are really the same thing, simply looked at from different perspectives.) In quantum mechanics gravity's transfer particle is called a graviton, and it moves at the speed of light.

The farther you move from a gravitational mass, the less its force will affect you.

The drop in the gravitational force is governed by what is known as the inverse square law, which says the attraction of any object drops in relation to the square of the distance you move from it. If you are floating over the surface of the planet and then move x times away from it, you will feel $1/x^2$ times less gravity. So if you move 10 times farther away from where you were, you will feel 1/100 the force gravity.

Fundamental Forces: Strong and Weak Nuclear Forces

The strong and weak nuclear forces are fundamental forces, but they were discovered much later than electromagnetism and gravity primarily because they only interact with matter at a subatomic level.

Strong nuclear force is the strongest of the four fundamental forces.

Strong nuclear force is 100 times stronger than the next strongest force, electromagnetism, and 1036 times the strength of the weakest force, gravity. That said, for the thousands of years people have studied physics, it never occurred to any one to even look for the strong force. That is because, despite the strong force's strength, it has such a limited range that it only interacts with matter across the distance of an atom's nucleus. In fact, its range is only about 10-15 meters, so small that the nuclei of the largest atoms—those filled with the highest number of protons and neutrons—are only just barely small enough for the strong force to keep working, making the nuclei of those atoms unstable.

The strong force was not discovered until the 1930s when scientists discovered the neutron.

Until that time atomic nuclei were thought to consist of a collection of protons and electrons grouped together in such a way that kept them mutually attracted. With the discovery of the neutron, however, a new force was needed to hold positively charged protons together with uncharged neutrons.

Strong Nuclear force interacts with Quarks.

The strong force actually does not interact directly with the protons and neutrons but with the fundamental particle that makes up protons and neutrons, quarks. Quarks come in three different color groupings: red, green and blue. (Quarks are not actually these colors; red, green and blue are just familiar names given to bits of matter that are utterly outside our experience as humans, to make them easier to comprehend.) The different colors of quarks combine to create protons and neutrons. Within each proton and neutron, the strong force holds the quarks together. That, in turn, bleeds out into the rest of the nucleus in a residual effect, holding the protons and neutrons together as well.

Like the other fundamental forces, the strong force is mediated at the quantum level using a transfer particle known as a gluon. However, unlike the transfer particles for gravity and electromagnetism (gravitons and photons, respectively), gluons have mass. It is the gluon's mass that limits the area where it can spread the strong force to only within the nucleus.

Weak nuclear force causes a type of radioactive decay.

The other fundamental force operating inside the nucleus is the weak force. The weak force causes a specific type of radioactive decay called beta decay, so named because it causes the decaying atom to emit a beta particle, which can be either an electron or a positron (a form of anti-mater also known as an anti-electron), as a by product of changing into a different element.

Several things happen at once during beta decay, and we should look at each one individually. We saw while looking at the strong force that an atom's protons and neutrons are made up of smaller, fundamental particles called quarks, and it is the quarks that actually interact with the strong force. As it turns out, quarks are the only particle that interacts with all four fundamental forces, which means that inside the nucleus they are interacting with the weak force as well.

Besides three different colors: red, blue and green, Quarks can be divided into six different flavors: up, down, charm, strange, top and bottom.

Before we get to how the weak force interacts with quarks, there is something else you should know about them. We mentioned above that quarks come in three different colors: red, blue and green. However, they also can be divided into six different flavors: up, down, charm, strange, top and bottom. (This makes 18 different possible combinations of quark, each with a color and a flavor.) Of these flavors only up and down quarks are stable enough to form protons and neutrons.

What the weak force does is switch up quarks to down quarks and down quarks to up quarks.

This is actually the only thing that the weak force does, but it has several effects. First since quarks join to produce protons and neutrons (two up quarks and one down quark make a proton, while two down and one up quark make a neutron), the sudden change of one type of quark to another changes that combination. β− decay is beta decay where change of quarks causes a neutron to become a proton. This also causes the atom to emit an electron and a electron antineutrino. β + decay is the opposite, where a proton changes to a neutron and the atom emits a positron and an electron neutrino.

In both cases the decaying atom changes into a different kind of atom. In general, beta decay takes place in unstable isotopes (atoms that have a different number of protons and neutrons) and stabilizes the nucleus by equalizing the ratio of these particles. For instance, beta decay will turn the unstable plutonium 15 into far more stable strontium 16.

Quantum Mechanics

Quantum mechanics is the study of quanta, the most basic individual unit of any substance.

Quantum mechanics first began as a discipline within physics in 1900 when Max Planck determined that energy radiated as heat could not just radiate at any temperature, but that it could only rise and fall—and thus be emitted or absorbed—at certain, set levels. (Think of it as the difference between stairs and ramps. Stairs have set spaces where you can stand and set spaces where you cannot. Planck said that raising energy levels such as temperature was akin to climbing a set of stairs one step at a time.)

Radiation that produces heat (and thus all electromagnetic radiation, including visible light) is made up of tiny little particles, which Planck named quanta from the Latin work "quantus," which means "how much."

Planck developed an equation to describe this situation, $E = h\nu$ in which ν stood for the already well known frequencies of electromagnetic spectrum (and which in 1900 was thought of as only acting like a wave), h stood for a number called the Planck constant that equaled 6.63×10^{-34} J s ("J s" is for Joule seconds), and E was the energy level for quanta of that frequency.

In 1905 Albert Einstein used Planck's work to define the photon, which is one quantum of electromagnetic radiation.

Photons are generally thought of as light, but only some energies of photons are visible. Photons can have any energy that corresponds to electromagnetic frequency, but instead of being a continuous wave, they are thought of as individual particles.

Waves and particles are the same thing look at in different ways.

The discovery of the particle aspect of a wave led to a realization that waves and particles were actually the same thing, looked at in different ways. This idea, called wave-particle duality, accounted for the centuries long debate between physicists over whether light was a wave or a particle, with each side producing compelling evidence to prove its thesis. As it turned out light—like everything in the universe—was both. This relationship was demonstrated by Louis de Broglie who developed the equation $p = h/\lambda$ showing that the Planck constant (h) divided by a particle's wavelength (λ, pronounced lambda) would equal its momentum (p). Since all particles are moving and have momentum, all particles have wavelengths.

One of the most important aspects of wave-particle duality comes from studying atoms.

The orbits of electrons around the atomic nuclei had at one time been thought to mimic the orbits of planets around the sun. Now, however, two important factors came into play to change that view. The first was the realization that electrons could only orbit at certain distances from the nucleus. When changing from one electron shell to the next, an electron would not take a gradual trajectory to its new home in the way a spaceship from Earth to Mars might. The electron would simply vanish from one shell and appear instantaneously at the next. In essence, electrons could also only display certain quanta of energy. They could have one energy level or another, but they could not exist in between.

The second important thing that quantum mechanics showed physicists is that "orbit" does not describe electrons and is only symbolic.

Since all particles are also waves, an electron could not simply be in one place at one time, but had to exist as across a range of areas as a frequency which described its momentum.

The Heisenberg uncertainty principle states you can measure the position of an electron or the velocity, but not both at once.

This seemingly nonsensical idea was explained mathematically though the Heisenberg uncertainty principle, which stated that it was possible to measure the exact position of a particle, and it was possible to measure the exact velocity of a particle, but you could not know both factors at once. In other words, measuring one would make it impossible to measure the other. This was an unavoidable fact of reality given de Broglie's equation; if you were moving you were spread out like a wave.

No particles in the universe can be said to have definite positions in space.

A strange side effect of this was it meant that no particles in the universe could be said to have definite positions in space. Instead, everything had a likely position given its velocity. Matter could not be said to exist at certain points in space, it could merely have certain probabilities of existing at those points.

Gravity is still a problem.

The 21st century understanding of gravity comes from Einstein's work on Special and General Relativity. The various predictions made by Einstein's theories have been proven correct experimentally on numerous occasions, and evidently his ideas accurately explain reality. However, they do not mix with quantum mechanics.

Physics has three zones which do not mix - relativity, quantum mechanics and Newtonian.

It is possible to look at physics and think of there as being three distinct zones: relativity, which describes the very big and the very fast; quantum mechanics, which describes the very small; and Newtonian physics, which describes everything in between.

But Newtonian physics easily unifies with quantum theory since the chaos and weirdness at the individual wave-particle level smooths out as you add more and more particles together, which is what we see when we look at the macro world in which we live. (That is, when you look at an object in front of you, you see it existing in a definite point in space because so many particles make it up the probability that they will all end suddenly existing elsewhere—the way individual particles can—drops to nearly zero.) Additionally, three of the four fundamental forces, electromagnetism, the strong force and the weak force, can all be explained through quantum mechanics using their three transfer particles; photons, gluons and bosons. They have been unified. However, the use of a gravity transfer particle, the graviton, in models has been less successful at bringing the experimentally accurate predictions of relativity in line with the functioning of reality at the quantum level.

States of Matter

Matter on Earth can exist in three main states or phases: solid, liquid and gas. There is also a fourth phase, plasma, that occurs when matter is superheated.

The primary difference between the different phases of matter is the behavior of molecules relative to the temperature the matter is exposed to. The lower the temperature, the closer together and more locked together the molecules are. The higher the temperature, the each other apart the molecules are, and the more they move relative to each other.

Solid

Solid matter exists in a state where its molecules are locked together in a rigid structure preventing them from moving and, as a result, solid matter is held together in a specific shape.

There are two primary types of solids, each defined by the structures in which their molecules are held. When the molecules in solid matter maintain a uniform organization they form a polycrystalline structure. This is how molecules in metal, ice and salt are organized. Polycrystalline structures are generally a result of the molecules' ionic properties. Water molecules, for instance, are formed in such a way that there are distinct ends, one with two hydrogen atoms and one with a single oxygen atom. The structure of the atoms within a water molecule means these ends are charged, giving it what amount to poles and causing water molecules to join only in specific patterns. Under a microscope polycrystalline solids are generally described as resembling lattice work or a chain link fence, with the same pattern of molecules from one end to the other.

When molecule's electromagnetic properties do not incline them to form into particular structures, they glob together in whatever patterns they can. This produces amorphous solids, most notably foams, glass and many types of plastic. Amorphous solids have no regular pattern throughout their structure and, as a result, are poor conductors of heat and electricity.

Liquid

When solids are heated past a certain point, the electromagnetic bonds holding their molecules together loosen, and the molecules are able to move more freely.

While the temperatures required for this to happen can vary widely, the particular physical qualities of a liquid are always the same. Liquids are considered to be fluids, which differ from solids primarily in their ability to take the shape of any container they are held in. This is the result of a less intense electromagnetic connection between the molecules than there is in solids; however, there is still enough, that liquids want to stay in the same place. This is why liquids still maintain a low density that is nearly identical to their densities in solid form, and why they will maintain a constant volume rather than just drift off the way gasses do.

Liquids also have a property known as viscosity, which describes their willingness to flow away from themselves. Liquids such as water and honey have a constant viscosity and are known as Newtonian fluids. Non-Newtonian fluids, such as a goopy mixture of water and cornstarch can change their viscosities.

Gas

The third state of matter that is commonly found on Earth is gas. Gasses are formed when matter is heated beyond its liquid state so that the electromagnetic bonds holding its molecules together are severed almost completely.

Gasses are also considered fluids and like liquids have no definite shape. But unlike liquids they lack a definite volume and have an extremely low density compared to their solid forms.

Since gasses lack both a shape and a volume, they will expand to fill any container they are placed in. Left unbounded they will expand forever. Conversely, gasses are perfectly happy to compress together in an enclosed space. (However, the more molecules of a gas that are enclosed in a space, the higher the gas's pressure—the force exerted by the molecules on the container's surface—will be.) One interesting thing about this expansion and compression is that it will always be homogeneous, meaning that as a gas expands to fill a container, there will never be pockets of higher density of molecules with pockets of lower density of molecules. The molecules will expand to fill the container equally.

Plasma

Plasma is the next step up from a gas; it is when a gas's molecules become super heated to the point where the molecular bonds themselves break down and the atoms begin shedding their electrons.

Although plasma is rarely found on Earth, it is the most common state of matter throughout the universe. (It is the primary state of matter in stars, for instance.) Plasma has some unique characteristics, not the least of which is that it is ionized, or electrically charged. In many ways plasma acts like a gas. It lacks any definite shape or volume, and it will homogeneously fill any container. However, it can also be manipulated by electromagnetic fields, which alters its shape or contains it. Plasma is a super-heated, magnetically charged gas.

Human Body Science (Anatomy and Physiology) Tutorials

Circulatory System

Tour of the System

The easiest way to see how the circulatory system works is by taking a tour with erythrocytes (red blood cells) through the system:

The erythrocytes start in the *left ventricle* of the heart.

They then move through the *aortic valve* into the *aorta*.

As the aorta branches into smaller arteries, the erythrocytes move into an *artery* then split into smaller blood vessels known as *arterioles*.

From arterioles, the erythrocytes pass into a capillary, or capillary bed.

Capillaries are tiny blood vessels and it is in these vessels that the exchange of oxygen, nutrients and carbon dioxide takes place.

After this exchange, the erythrocytes are de-oxygenated (oxygen has been removed from the erythrocyte).

Blood that contains these de-oxygenated erythrocytes is also known as *venous blood*.

The erythrocytes, which now contain carbon dioxide and other waste products, pass from the capillaries into *venules*.

Venules come together to form veins.

From the veins, the erythrocytes flow into the superior vena cava, and into the right atrium. They pass through the tricuspid valve into the right ventricle.

The erythrocytes pass through the pulmonary valve and into the pulmonary artery on their way to the lungs. The pulmonary artery is the only artery that carries deoxygenated blood.

In the lungs, the erythrocytes give up their carbon dioxide and absorb oxygen. Now the blood goes back to the left atrium, through the mitral valve and into the left ventricle, ready to start its journey once again.

The movement of the blood to and from the heart is the systemic circulation and the movement of the blood from the heart to the lungs and back again is the pulmonary circulation.

The blood pressure in arteries is regulated by muscular contraction or expansion of the arterial walls, according to need.

The circulatory system also consists of the lymphatic system, which has the job of distributing lymph throughout the body. This is how lymph moves through the system:

In capillaries, the serum, or the liquid part of the blood, seeps through the tissues.

If tissues are inflamed, the capillaries are more permeable and so seepage is faster.

This serum is called lymph.

Lymph makes its way through tissues, until it collects in the lymphatic ducts.

Once in the ducts, lymph begins to make its way back to the venous blood stream.

As lymph moves, lymph nodes filtered it.

These lymph nodes contain leukocytes (white blood cells) which are ready to attack bacteria or viruses.

Functions

The circulatory system has several key functions, including:

- Controlling the movement of blood and lymph through the body

- Exchanging gases (oxygen and carbon dioxide) with other cells and tissues in the body

- Exchanging nutrients (such as amino acids and electrolytes) with other cells and tissues

- Helping with immune responses

- Helping with clotting

- Helping in the maintenance of body temperature and pH (maintaining homeostasis)

Components

Heart: This is what pumps blood around the body. Because the heart is a muscle, it also needs oxygen, so it has its own circulatory system known as the *coronary circulation*, which takes blood to and from the heart.

Aorta: This is the main artery that receives blood from the heart. It is a very tough, muscular artery.

Arteries: These blood vessels also contain muscle to make them elastic. This helps to move the blood along.

Arterioles: Also muscular these smaller vessels contract to deliver blood to the capillaries.

Capillaries: These are the diameter of a single cell, making exchange of gases and other products from erythrocytes easy.

Venules: Many of these small blood vessels come together to form a vein.

Veins: Unlike arteries, these do not contract. With a tube-like structure, they contain valves to prevent blood from flowing backwards.

Lymph ducts: These empty lymph into the veins.

Lymph nodes: These act as filters for the lymph and are very important in the immune system. Inflammation of these usually shows infection in the body.

Common Diseases and Disorders

Angina: Is a type of chest pain that often radiates down the arm. Angina is caused when the heart cannot receive the blood and oxygen that it needs (usually because the coronary arteries are blocked with plaque).

Cardiac Arrest: The heart stops pumping blood around the body. Unlike a heart attack, this can happen suddenly without a known cause (such as coronary heart disease).

Coronary heart disease: Coronary arteries (which supply the heart with blood) are narrowed because of plaque deposits on their walls. These deposits prevent enough oxygen from reaching the heart.

Heart Attack or Myocardial Infarction: When the coronary arteries (which supply blood the heart muscle with blood) become blocked with plaque, blood flow to the heart muscles is reduced. This causes damage to the heart muscle as well as increasing the risk of part of the heart muscle dying.

Phlebitis: This is inflammation of a vein. A common place is in the legs, where the veins swell and block the blood, so the leg swells markedly.

Varicose veins: Unnaturally swollen veins caused by faulty valves. These are usually in the legs.

Medical Terminology

Blood pressure: This is how much pressure there is against the walls of the main arteries. The systolic pressure is when the ventricles of the heart contract and the diastolic pressure is when ventricles relax and refill. The classic blood pressure measurement is 120/80 (120 is the systole value and 80 is the diastole value).

Erythrocytes: These red blood cells carry oxygen, carbon dioxide and other products through the circulatory system.

Hypertension: High blood pressure

Hypotension: Low blood pressure

Leukocytes: There are several different kinds of white blood cells and they play a key role in the immune system.

Platelets: Platelets are cell fragments found in the blood. They are essential for blood clotting.

Pulse rate/heart rate: The number of times the heart beats per minute.

The circulatory system is also important when *assessing a person's color*. The color changes when a greater or lesser quantity of blood diverts to the skin, so color is a good indicator of health.

Terms to denote a lack of color include: pale, ashen, pallid, sallow, white, colorless, white as a ghost, blanched.

Terms to denote too much color include: florid, flushed, crimson, ruddy, feverish.

There are also *trauma terms* for the circulatory system:

Bleeding: Blood coming from a lesion. Internal bleeding is bleeding inside the body, often caused by an injury or disease. Blood may sometimes leak from an opening such as the mouth or anus.

Bleeding nose (Epistaxis): Blood coming from the nose, usually due to trauma. A bleeding nose can sometimes start spontaneously due to increased blood pressure.

Bruised: Discolored due to a blow. Usually the skin is not broken (a bruise is also called a contusion).

Cut or Incision: A clean-cut wound or slit such as one caused by a knife.

Crush: Caused by pressure a crush is a contusion or bruise, showing internal bleeding.

Gash or laceration: A wound that is torn or ragged.

Scrape: An abrasion or graze caused by scraping off the upper tissues of the skin.

Swollen: Bigger than usual, often through accumulation of fluid.

Throbbing: When used with pain, it means that the pain gets worse in a rhythmic pattern (with the heartbeat).

Other miscellaneous medical and trauma terms include:

Blood blister: A dark swelling of the skin caused by pinching, which breaks a small blood vessel. The skin remains unbroken.

Blood tests: A variety of tests carried out with a blood sample. A blood test can check for many disorders including anemia, infections or even liver damage.

Blood in the urine: Shows problems with the bladder, kidneys or prostate gland.

Hemangioma (blood spot or birthmark): Is a dark red discoloration of the skin.

Occult blood: "Occult" means hidden. To detect colon cancer, feces is checked for occult blood.

Palpitations or bumping: This refers to an irregular heartbeat, often experienced by the patient as a "bumping in the chest."

Tarry stools: These are feces that dark in color, like tar, caused by old blood in the digestive tract. Tarry stools can show internal bleeding.

Transfusion: Transfusing, or giving of blood taken from a blood donor.

The Digestive System

Tour of the System

The digestive system is an extensive system that begins at the lips and ends at the anus. The easiest way to explore the digestive system is on a journey with a peanut butter and jelly sandwich (PB&J):

The PB&J passes through the lips and into the mouth (oral cavity).

The oral cavity contains teeth and the tongue. Beneath the tongue is the floor of the mouth and above the tongue, the hard palate.

The soft palate (which does not contain bone) is at the back of the mouth.

The PB&J is *masticated* (chewed) by the teeth.

There are normally 32 teeth and in each arch there are:

- 4 incisors

- 2 cuspids (or canines - they resemble the long cuspids that dogs have)

- 4 premolars or bicuspids

- 6 molars. The last molar is the "wisdom tooth."

Chewing the PB&J also requires assistance from the muscular tongue.

Chewing stimulates the release of saliva from the salivary glands in the mouth to moisten the sandwich. Saliva contains enzymes that help to break down carbohydrates.

The PB&J is now a homogeneous smooth mass called a bolus.

Swallowing or deglutition is a complex process controlled by the nervous system.

The lingual nerve in the tongue determines when the bolus is 'ready' for swallowing.

Once the bolus is pushed to the back of the tongue, receptors start the pharyngeal phase of swallowing.

This phase is when breathing, chewing, coughing and other activities stop.

The bolus passes the tonsils, the pharynx and goes into the esophagus to the stomach.

The stomach is located just below the diaphragm and when empty it has a volume of around 45 ml. When full, it can extend to hold as much as three liters of food.

In the stomach, the bolus mixes with liquids, acid and digestive juices.

These break the bolus down into simpler chemical substances so they can be absorbed into the blood more easily.

After some hours, the semi-liquid mass, now called chyme, passes into the small intestine.

In the first part of the small intestine, called the duodenum, bile from the liver emulsifies fats. Pancreatic juice and enzymes also break down materials further.

Broken down materials are absorbed into the bloodstream and taken to the liver for filtration, toxin removal and further processing.

Anything remaining in the small intestine moves to the large intestine via peristalsis.

Fermentation, aided by gut bacteria left in the chyme, breaks down some of the remaining substances.

The chyme moves into the cecum, which is a pouch that connects the last part of the small intestine (ileum) with the first part of the large intestine.

Attached to the cecum is the appendix. In humans, the appendix is vestigial, which means it has no known function.

The large intestine takes around 16 hours to complete the digestive processes.

Digested matter moves from the cecum to the colon.

The colon is able to absorb vitamins (including vitamin K) produced by the bacteria which inhabit the colon (colonic bacteria).

The colon also absorbs salts and water and stores feces until defecation.

Feces move along the colon by peristalsis to the last part of the large intestine, the rectum.

From here, defecation, the final process of digestion occurs.

This whole process of digestion takes between 24 and 72 hours.

Functions

The main function of the digestive system is to digest, or break down food into smaller chemical components (also called *catabolism*).

Components

Pharynx

This is the part of the throat located behind the mouth and nasal cavity.

Tongue

This muscle is used to manipulate food during chewing (mastication). The tongue also contains taste buds.

Esophagus

This is a muscular tube connecting the pharynx to the stomach. A bolus moves through the esophagus via peristalsis.

Epiglottis

This is a cartilage flap attached at the entrance to the voice box (larynx). When this is closed, it prevents food from entering the trachea (windpipe).

Large intestine

This starts at the cecum, contains the colon and ends at the rectum. It is involved in absorbing some nutrients but primarily water and salts.

Small intestine

Most digestion and absorption occurs in the small intestine and this is why this organ is very long, offering the maximum surface area for its digestive functions.

Stomach

This is J shaped and connects the esophagus to the small intestine. As well as a food mixing and processing area, the stomach also 'holds' food until it is ready to move into the small intestine. The stomach is acidic as its enzymes work best at a low pH.

Liver

The liver produces several chemicals needed for digestion. It is also able to store some nutrients such as vitamins.

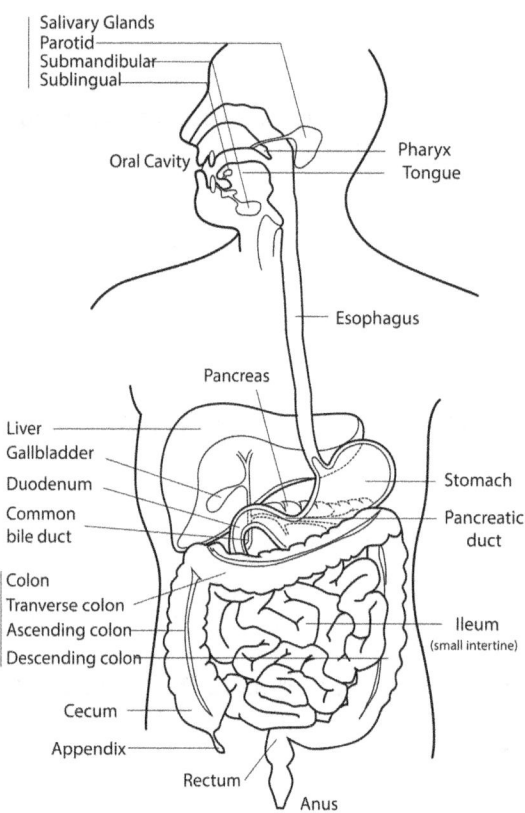

Pancreas

This produces several digestive juices to help in digestion.

Gallbladder

This produces and stores bile until required by the small intestine.

Rectum

The final part of the large intestine it temporarily stores feces.

Common Diseases and Disorders

Appendicitis: This is inflammation or infection of the appendix. If infected the appendix can swell and burst. Also called peritonitis, this is very serious because then the contents of the intestines spill into the abdominal cavity.

Colon cancer: This can develop without symptoms, which is why doctors often take an occult blood sample every two years. This test detects small amounts of blood in the feces, which can be a symptom of colon cancer.

Constipation: Refers to infrequent or difficult evacuation of the feces.

Diarrhea: Is abnormal frequency and liquidity of feces.

Diverticulosis: As people age, the large intestine sometimes forms small pouches. Sometimes sharp foods like seeds or grains lodge in these pouches and cause inflammation or infection. This is diverticulitis.

Gallstones: Hard stones created from a buildup of bile in the gall bladder. They cause acute pain but are often able to be removed with a catheter and ultrasound.

Perforated ulcer: A stomach ulcer has broken through the stomach wall is now perforated. This allows the contents of the stomach to move into the abdominal cavity and can be very serious.

A 'sore mouth' could mean one of many things, including cold sores (herpes simplex), mouth ulcers (aphthous ulcers) or lesions of the teeth and gums.

Sore throat are another common problem, usually due to infection in the tonsils, or an inflamed pharynx.

Stomach ulcers: Prolonged chronic stress is often the main cause of stomach ulcers. Because the stomach produces too much stomach acid, it damages the mucosal covering of the stomach, causing a lesion.

Medical Terminology

GI tract: Gastrointestinal or GI tract can sometimes include all structures from the mouth to the anus, but medically it is often differentiated between the upper and lower GI tracts.

Lower GI: The lower gastrointestinal tract includes the large intestine, small intestine and anus.

Peristalsis: This is a very strong, rhythmic contraction and relaxation of muscles throughout the digestive system that push the contents along.

Upper GI: The upper GI or gastrointestinal tract generally refers to the esophagus, stomach and duodenum.

The Endocrine System

Tour of the System

The endocrine system is an amazingly complex system with many important roles throughout the body. It works alongside the nervous system to coordinate functions of of the different body systems.

The endocrine system contains endocrine glands that release their products (known as hormones) directly into the bloodstream.

Hormones are substances that arouse the body into activity. Hormones are often dependent on one another in their action. That is, the secretion of one hormone will often excite another gland to produce its hormone too. The balance that the body strikes with these hormones is unique for each individual.

Although hormones travel around the body in the bloodstream, they only affect certain cells, which are their target cells. Only target cells will contain the correct molecular information that will allow a hormone to bind to that particular cell.

How cells respond to hormones depends on the cell itself as well as the hormone. One hormone may synthesize (make) a product in one type of cell and make a completely different product in another type of cell.

The easiest way, when touring this complex system, is to look at where endocrine glands are and what hormones they secrete.

The diagrams below show endocrine glands and their hormones.

HUMAN BODY SCIENCE

Hormones produced in the head and neck

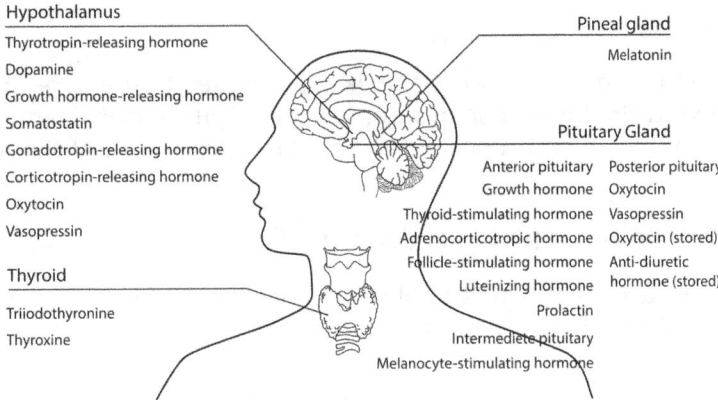

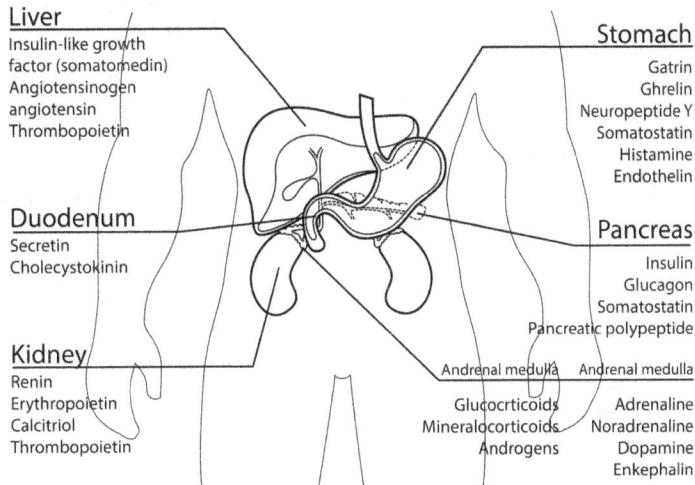

Functions

The endocrine system secretes hormones into the bloodstream to regulate the body, helping to maintain homeostasis.

Components

Hypothalamus

This is the 'master' endocrine gland, located in the brain. The hypothalamus links the endocrine and nervous system. The hypothalamus receives information about pain, stress etc. It also regulates the autonomic nervous system that controls body temperature, hunger, thirst etc. The hypothalamus regulates the release of several hormones that act on other glands.

The pituitary gland

The pituitary gland is in the center of the skull, attached to the hypothalamus. The hypothalamus controls the release or suppression of pituitary hormones. As well as having its own unique effects, it can influence the performance of the other endocrine glands.

It has two parts, a posterior pituitary gland and the anterior pituitary gland.

The posterior pituitary gland tends to store oxytocin, used for uterine contractions and anti-diuretic hormone (ADH), which stimulates water retention.

Hormones released from the *anterior pituitary gland*

Hormone group	Function	Example	How it works
Somatotrophs	Stimulate the thyroid gland.	Growth hormone (GH)	If growth hormone is produced for too long, gigantism occurs. If growth hormone is produced after the epiphyseal disks have calcified in the skeleton, acromegaly occurs, causing abnormally large hands, feet and mandible (jaw). If not enough growth hormone is produced, the child will not grow and artificial growth hormone is usually administered to correct this.
Thyrotrophs	These hormones stimulate activity in other glands.	Thyroid-stimulating hormone (TSH)	This controls secretion of other hormones in the thyroid gland.
Gonadotrophs	These are involved in ovulation, although they are present in both males and females.	Follicle stimulating hormone (FSH) and luteinizing hormone (LH)	FSH and LH are needed to secrete estrogens and progesterone and assists in reproduction,

Lactotrophs	Lactotrophs are involved in growth and regulation of mammary glands.	Prolactin	Initiates milk production in mammary glands
Corticotrophs	Synthesize ACTH	Adrenocor-ticot-rophin (ACTH)	ACTH stimulates the adrenal cortex to produce glucocorticoids (required in glucose metabolism).

There are also several other hormones secreted from the pituitary gland.

The Thyroid gland

Situated at the base of the larynx, its middle part, the isthmus, covers the second and third cartilaginous rings of the trachea.

It secretes the thyroid hormones thyroxin and triiodothyronine. These have an important role in controlling metabolism (including energy or ATP production) throughout the body.

It also secretes calcitonin that alters calcium levels in the blood.

The Parathyroid glands

There are usually four parathyroid glands, two on each side of the thyroid gland. Although they are very small, they control the quantity of calcium and magnesium in the blood stream.

Without them, there is not enough calcium in the blood for the nervous system to function properly. Those who have *hyperparathyroidism* have de-mineralized bones and the calcium in their bones is urinated away.

Adrenal or Suprarenal glands

These are located on the top of the kidneys. The adrenal glands produce three types of steroids. *Steroid* hormones are fat (lipid) hormones.

The exterior of the adrenal glands (*adrenal cortex*) produces three types of hormones:

- **Mineralocorticoids** - control sodium and potassium levels in the body

- **Glucocorticoids** – involved in metabolism and resistance to stress. One of these is cortisone, a hormone that has a variety of functions in the body

- **Androgens** – These have little effect on the body as significant amounts of androgens are produced in the testes. In women, these contribute to sex drive.

The inner of the adrenal glands, the *adrenal medulla* produces **epinephrine** and **norepinephrine** (noradrenalin). These hormones prepare the body to either "fight or flight." Epinephrine (adrenalin) increases the heart rate and breathing rate, adjusts blood supply to the extremities and causes the blood to clot more readily. Therefore, if you are suddenly startled, you notice these changes in the body.

Pancreas

The pancreas contains special cells called *islets of Langerhans*. These secrete several hormones:

Insulin - controls the amount of glucose in the blood stream. Insulin causes removal and storage of glucose from the blood.

Glucagon – Raises blood sugar levels by breaking down glycogen in the liver. This causes the release of glucose into the blood.

The other two hormones, **somatostatin** and **pancreatic polypeptides** assist insulin and glucagon with their actions.

Pineal gland

This gland is located in the brain and secretes **melatonin,** a hormone that play an important role in the sleep and wake cycle. The cause of jet lag is through melatonin disruption.

Thymus gland

This plays a key role in immunity, helping white blood cells to mature.

There are also hormones produced throughout other tissues and organs in the body, including erythropoietin from the kidney, which helps to increase the rate of erythrocyte (red blood cell) production.

Common Diseases and Disorders

Cretinism: Caused by a lack of thyroid hormones produced during development. The severe hormone deficiency causes a hard form of edema, called myxedema.

Diabetes: An insufficiency of insulin production causes diabetes. For those who suffer from type 1 diabetes, it means that the cells in their pancreas have stopped producing insulin, or produce very little. Those with Type 2 diabetes are able to produce some insulin, but not enough to regulate blood glucose levels. Type 2 diabetes is often seen in obese patients.

Goiter: This is an enlargement of the thyroid gland, often caused by iodine deficiency.

Hyperthyroidism: Is caused by too much thyroxin, resulting in a higher than normal metabolic rate.

Hypothyroidism: Is a lack of thyroxin.

Polycystic ovary syndrome: This is a common female endocrine disorder. Although it may have genetic causes, hormone imbalances play a key role in this syndrome.

Medical Terminology

Autonomic nervous system: This is part of the nervous system. It helps to control the body. It is usually unconscious and controls actions such as the heart rate, digestion and respiratory rate.

Endocrinology: Is the study of the endocrine system and the resulting hormone balance.

Homeostasis: This is the ability of the human body to maintain a stable internal environment, when dealing with both internal and external environmental changes.

Negative feedback: Helps to maintain homeostasis in the body. If a gland is producing too much of one hormone, signals are sent to the brain and an opposing hormone is released. This reduces the levels of the first hormone. For example, glucagon and insulin, regulating blood glucose levels.

Positive feedback: Rarely seen in the body, a positive feedback loop is the secretion of oxytocin during delivery. This increases contractions to allow delivery of the baby.

The Integumentary System

Tour of the System

The integumentary system is composed of the skin, hair and nails. It has a variety of functions, but the main one is to protect the body. It is the largest organ system in the body, consisting of around 15% of the total body weight.

The skin is a key indicator of an individual's health status. It is readily visible, without any intrusive procedures. The skin of the face and hands can reveal a lot about the circulatory system, the lifestyle of the patient and their general health. Those who have yellowing skin are usually suffering from jaundice whereas those who have a blue-grey tint are suffering from cyanosis. A deep red hue could show hypertension (high blood pressure) or white skin can be an indicator of medical shock. How skin feels can also show disease or trauma. Skin may feel cold, clammy, hot or dry.

Functions

The skin **protects internal tissues and organs.**

The skin **prevents organisms** (such as bacteria or viruses) from entering the body.

The skin **protects the body from dehydrating.**

The skin **acts as a waterproof barrier**. It allows a wet body to exist in dry air, allows immersion in fresh water without swelling with water, or immersion in salt water without becoming desiccated.

The skin **protects the body from sudden temperature changes** (maintains homeostasis). On hot days, the skin helps regulate body temperature in three main ways:

Arterioles vasodilate and send more blood to superficial capillaries in the skin. This allows heat loss.

The hairs on the skin remain flat, preventing the insulating air from becoming trapped between the hairs and the skin.

Sweating or perspiration is also essential for cooling the body, through the process of evaporation.

The skin **protects the body from UV damage** by secreting melanin. Pigmented or freckled skin is an adaptation to intense sunlight.

The skin **excretes waste materials**, such as salts and urea, through perspiration.

The skin **stores a variety of substances** include water, fat, glucose and vitamin D.

The skin **produces Vitamin D** from UV exposure. An absence of Vitamin D causes rickets.

The skin **forms new skin cells** to repair skin damage.

The skin **maintains the form** of the body.

The **skin acts as a receptor** for:

- touch

- pressure

- pain
- heat
- cold

These receptors are also parts of the *somatosensory system*. Because the skin receives many stimuli, it plays a major role in man's adaptation to his environment. In particular, the skin acts as an early warning system for unhealthy conditions.

Components

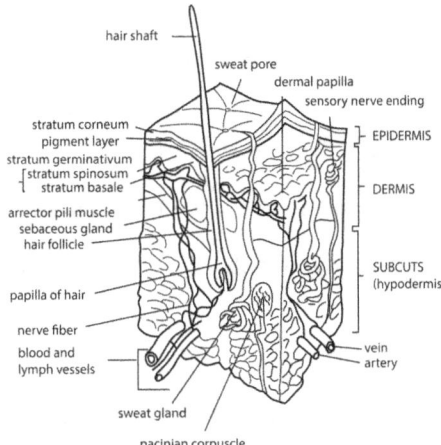

Skin consists of two main layers, the epidermis and the dermis and these contain several other components:

The Epidermis

This is the top layer of skin made up of epithelial cells.

The cells lower in the epidermis are responsible for the growth of this layer. As mitosis (cell division) occurs at the *basale layer,* cells move up through the strata (thin layer), pushed upwards by the dividing cells below.

The epidermis does not contain blood vessels.

There are several different types of cell found in the epidermis, including keratinocytes and melanocytes.

Keratinocytes are the most common cell found in the epidermis.

Keratinocytes mainly act as a barrier cell. They also produce a protein known as *keratin.*

Keratin makes the top layer strong and water resistant.

As production of keratin increases, the keratinocytes die, called *cornification.*

These cornified keratinocytes are then lost (or shed) from the surface of the skin and replaced with new cells.

Renewal of the epidermis, also known as the process of maturation and desquamation takes around 21 days.

Nails develop in the epidermis and extend down into the dermis.

The Dermis

This contains a variety of connective tissues such as collagen and elastin that give skin stretch and flexibility.

The dermis helps cushion the body from stresses.

Ends of blood vessels and nerves are located in the dermis.

The blood vessels nourish and remove waste from the dermis and the basale layer of the epidermis.

The base of sweat glands and sebaceous glands are also located in the dermis.

Hair follicles may extend down into the underlying connective tissue, but they originally arise from the epidermis.

Sweat glands

Sweat glands are small tubular structures of the skin that produce sweat.

Eccrine sweat glands are all over the body. These play a key role in perspiring and cooling the skin

Apocrine sweat glands are larger and limited to the armpits and perianal areas. These become active during puberty and secrete odorous sweat.

Hair

The functions of hair include warmth and protection. In animals, hair has many other important functions such as camouflage.

Hair develops from keratin and it grows from the hair follicles that arise from the epidermis.

Once hair leaves the follicle, it is 'dead'.

Attached to the hair follicle is a sebaceous gland that lubricates the hair and the *erector pili* muscle that cause hair to stand up (goose bumps).

Nails

Nails protect the delicate fingertip from injury and help with delicate finger movements.

The condition of nails is also a good indicator of general health.

A nail consists of a nail plate, nail matrix and nail bed.

Nail plate cells grow in the *cell matrix* and push older nail plate cells forward.

The nail plate is the actual nail and this is made of keratin, forming a strong flexible material composed of layers of dead cells.

The *nail bed* is similar in structure to the skin, containing a dermis and epidermis.

Hypodermis

The *hypodermis* or *subcutaneous layer* is often associated with the skin. Its main function is to attach the skin to bone and muscle and supply the skin with blood vessels and nerves.

The main cells contained within the hypodermis are fibroblasts, macrophages and adipocytes (fat cells).

The hypodermis contains 50% of body fat and is essential as padding and insulation for the body.

Common Diseases and Disorders

Allergic reactions: The skin will often respond with a red rash due to exposure to an allergen. An allergen can be swallowed, inhaled, injected or even touched. Common allergens include, stings and animal fur.

Boil: A boil or furuncle develops from bacterial infection of the hair follicle.

Carcinomas: This is the medical term for cancer. The skin is subject to several kinds of carcinomas: basal cell, squamous cell carcinomas, as well as melanomas.

- Basal cell carcinoma is the most common type of skin cancer. Although it rarely kills, it is considered malignant as it can cause a lot of damage as it invades surrounding tissues.

- Squamous cell carcinoma is also a common cancer and can develop on the skin and other parts of the body. The cells involved in this type of carcinoma continue to divide uncontrollably.

A melanoma is a malignant tumor made up of melanocyte cells (which produce the pigment melanin). Many melanomas are visible as changes to existing moles or the appearance of a new lesion on the skin.

Cysts: If a sebaceous gland is blocked, a cyst can form. Because a cyst is enclosed, when it grows it displaces other structures around it. It does not invade other tissues (noninvasive).

Dermatitis: Sometimes used interchangeably with eczema. Dermatitis is inflammation of the skin of which there are several causes. Contact dermatitis often occurs on the hands as a reaction to latex gloves or chemicals.

Eczema: This condition has scaly, itchy patches with blisters.

Impetigo: A contagious bacterial infection of the skin that is very common amongst children

Pimples: When sebaceous glands are blocked, their oily discharge (sebum) accumulates under the skin, causing a small swelling. These often become infected.

Psoriasis: This is a skin disorder characterized by scaly red patches of the skin. When this disorder affects the fingers, it can cause nails to become deformed.

Pustules: These are common in acne. Pustules are small, inflamed and pus-filled lesions on the surface of the skin. They can occur anywhere on the body but are common on the face, shoulders and back.

Rash: Allergic reactions and several illnesses manifest with a skin rash. Nearly all "childhood diseases" such as measles and chicken pox have a skin rash. With these types of disease, often the rash provides the final diagnosis, even before the bacterial analyses are completed.

Medical Terminology

Basale layer: The lowest layer of the epidermis, this is the layer where epidermal cell division occurs.

Cyanosis: Also called 'blue disease,' this is a discoloration of the skin caused by low oxygen levels in tissues near the surface of the skin.

Homeostasis: This is the ability of the human body to maintain a stable internal environment, when dealing with both internal and external environmental changes.

Keratin: This protein has several functions in the skin, including, waterproofing.

Keratinocytes: These cells produce keratin.

Melanin: The pigment found in skin and hair that are the primary determinants of color.

Melanocytes: These cells produce melanin.

Vasodilation: This is when smooth muscle, found in arteries, arterioles and large veins relaxes to allow an increased flow of blood through. This plays an important role in controlling body temperature.

Vasoconstriction: The opposite of vasodilation, this occurs when blood vessels narrow, restricting the quantity of blood that can flow through these vessels.

The Reproductive System

Tour of the System

Reproduction is any type of reproduction that conceives a child and the reproductive systems of both males and females are required for conception to occur.

Under normal circumstances, an embryo will form when a spermatozoa (gamete) fertilizes a female ovum (a gamete). Gametes are different to other cells in the body because they only contain half of the usual numbers of chromosomes (which contain the genetic information). Each gamete contains 23 chromosomes (including sex chromosomes) and when they join a zygote is formed, containing 46 (or 23 pairs) of chromosomes. This zygote then develops into an embryo.

Because the ovum always contains one female sex (X) chromosome, the spermatozoa dictates the sex of the unborn child. The sperm cell may contain another X chromosome (producing a girl) or a Y chromosome that will produce a male child.

The fundamental organ of both reproductive systems is the gonad. In adult females, these are the ovaries and in adult males, the testes.

In the embryo, the gonads are at first undifferentiated and it is impossible to see whether it is male or female. With time, the gonads differentiate and certain features develop, while other features are suppressed. This is probably due to the influence of environmental conditions such as hormone production.

Hormones are critical for development and regulation of the reproductive system and there are many different types of hormones involved. During puberty in girls, the pituitary gland (located at the back of the brain) releases various hormones. These hormones signal the ovaries to release an ovum every twenty-eight days as well as inducing the ovary to start functioning as an endocrine (hormone releasing) gland itself.

The first hormone that the ovaries produce is estrogen. Estrogen induces the development of the secondary sexual characteristics (growth of breasts, change of body shape etc.). A second hormone, progesterone, produced by the corpus luteum encourages the endometrium to thicken, so that if fertilization occurs, the ovum will have the best conditions to grow there.

There is a similar development process in boys. The hormones released from the pituitary gland cause development of secondary sexual characteristics (facial hair, pubic hair, penis growth etc.) and development of the reproductive organs. The key male androgen is testosterone and this is important for normal sperm development as well as physical and mental well being in men.

Female Reproductive System

When the ovum (or gamete) develops in the ovary, it is in an ovarian follicle (sac).

The ovum moves along the fallopian tube towards the uterus with the help of contractions.

As the ovum matures, the follicular sac ruptures. The ruptured sac closes after releasing the egg and forms the corpus luteum. This produces the hormone progesterone.

The corpus luteum grows for about two weeks and then dies, unless it receives a different hormone from a developing embryo.

In pregnancy, however, the corpus luteum develops for several months and becomes large until the placenta takes over its job.

If during this journey, the ovum meets a sperm, fertilization may occur.

Fertilization often occurs in the fallopian tube although it can be in the uterus.

Once an ovum is fertilized, it is a zygote.

The zygote usually makes its way into the uterus and attaches to the special lining of the uterus called the endometrium and begins to develop into an embryo.

In a sexually mature woman, (before the menopause), this lining thickens up, becomes engorged with blood and is shed every twenty-eight days through menstruation.

The key time for fertilization is around halfway through the ovulation cycle and menstruation cannot occur if fertilization has occurred.

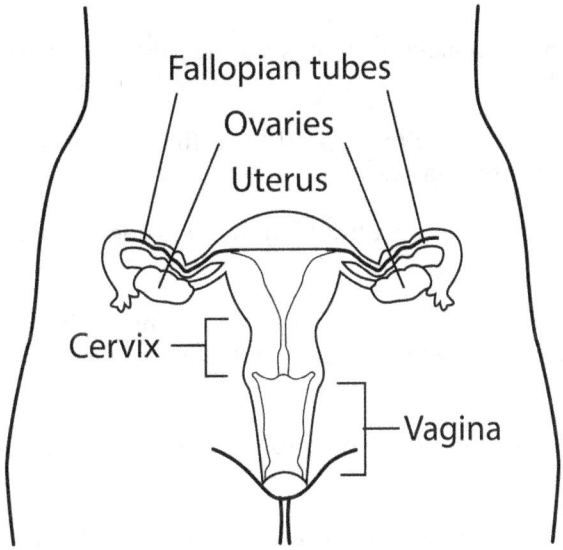

Male Reproductive System

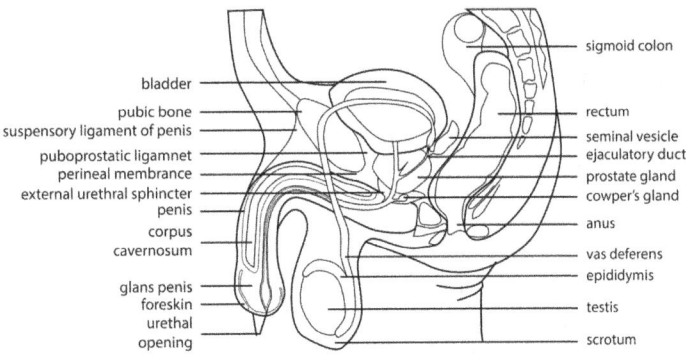

The male reproductive system consists of two main organs, the testes and the penis. There are also various glands and complicated tubal systems.

The testes make and store sperm cells (spermatozoa).

Three main glands lubricate the male reproductive system and nourish the spermatozoa.

One of these, the seminal vesicle produces the energy source that spermatozoa require for movement (motility).

The second, the bulbourethral glands produce a fluid released into the urethra. This helps in nourishing the spermatozoa.

Spermatozoa move to the third and final gland, the prostate gland, which produces the fluid vehicle (semen).

Semen is a mix of sperm cells, prostate fluid and seminal fluid. It also contains an enzyme, hyaluronidase, which helps the spermatozoa with penetrating the outer covering of the ovum.

From the prostate gland, semen moves into the urethra for expulsion during ejaculation.

Once ejaculation has occurred, sperm then travels through the vagina, towards the cervix and into the uterus or fallopian tubes to fertilize the ovum.

Functions

Since there are differences between males and females, reproduction creates a greater combination of genetic material in the offspring (child).

Female Components

Fallopian tube (or oviducts)

The two fallopian tubes connect to the uterus. They also have special properties that helps ova to move towards the uterus.

Uterus

This is the organ in which the embryo and then fetus develops during gestation. The uterus stays in place with the help of ligaments. The cervix of the uterus protrudes into the vagina. The uterus also plays an important part in the female sexual response, by diverting blood to the external genitalia.

Ovary

The ovaries produce the ovum (or gametes). Females have two, although they function independently. Ligaments attach the ovaries to the uterus, rather than to the fallopian tubes.

Vagina

The vagina is a flattened tube and serves as a sheath for the male organ in sexual intercourse. It opens to the exterior through two folds of skin, the labia majora, and the labia minora. At the anterior end of these folds is the clitoris, which is analogous to the head of the male penis. In fact, it has a common embryonic origin.

Male Components

Testes

These have two functions, production of spermatozoa and production of the male sex hormone, testosterone. The release of other hormones stimulates the production of both of these. The scrotum protects the testes and these are outside the body as spermatozoa function better at a temperature slightly lower than normal body temperature.

Penis

One of the main male sex organs it also carries urine from the bladder. The penis contains erectile tissue so that when it fills with blood an erection can occur. The penis needs to be erect for ejaculation to occur.

Common Diseases and Disorders

Amenorrhea: Is an absence of the menstrual cycle, caused by starvation, stress, major illness, as well as pregnancy.

Dysmenorrhea: These are severe symptoms of menstruation. During menstruation, it is usual for a woman to have stomach cramps, headaches and salt retention and if these affect daily living, it becomes dysmenorrhea.

Ectopic pregnancy: This is when a zygote attaches to the wall of the fallopian tube and begins to develop. It can also occur in the cervix, ovaries or abdomen.

Prostate cancer: This is one of the most common types of cancer in men, often diagnosed when men have difficulties with urinating.

Medical Terminology

Andrology: This is the branch of medicine for male reproductive health and urology.

Androgen: An androgen is any hormone that stimulates or maintains male characteristics, such as testosterone.

Artificial insemination (AI) or **Assisted Reproductive Technology**: This allows conception of a child without sexual intercourse/natural insemination.

Gestation: The length of time from fertilization until birth, around forty weeks in humans.

Menopause: This is when the ovaries no longer release ova and menstruation occur. This cessation is hormone-regulated. The formal date of menopause is from the time of the last menstruation, or period.

Obstetrics: This is the branch of medical care specifically for the female reproductive system, including pregnancy, birth and after birth (antenatal).

Ovulation: The point at which the ovum is released from the follicle sac.

Urethra: In men, the urethra carries both semen and urine out through the penis and in women; it carries urine from the bladder to the body exit.

The Respiratory System

Tour of the System

Life itself depends on the ability of the blood to deliver oxygen to and remove carbon dioxide from every cell, tissue and organ of the body. This is the responsibility of the respiratory system. This system also works very closely with other body systems, including the circulatory system.

The medulla in the brain regulates the **breathing rate**, based on the carbon dioxide content of the blood. Breathing is automatic, although under 'normal' conditions, there is the ability to alter the breathing rate consciously. The respiratory system consists of two main processes, **inhalation** and **exhalation,** which occurs in the **thoracic cavity**.

There is around 21% oxygen inhaled from the air and around 16% oxygen exhaled; this is why resuscitation can be effective in saving lives.

Inhalation

The diaphragm (located at the base of the rib cage) contracts, ribs move outwards and upwards, creating more space in the pleural cavity (space between the lining and covering of the lung). This changes the air pressure via a vacuum mechanism, forcing air into the lungs.

The air enters the nose through the *nostrils* (nares).

In the nasal cavity, air passes through *nasal conchae*.

The nasal conchae are mucosal tissues in the nose. As well as directing the movement of air, they heat, moisten and filter the air.

The air then passes through the *pharynx*, *larynx* and into the *trachea*.

The trachea is *ciliated* and secretes *mucus*.

Mucus is required to keep the airways lubricated and trap foreign particles, such as bacteria.

The cilia move mucus steadily upwards, until it can be swallowed and pass through the digestive system.

As the trachea moves towards the lungs, it divides into two main branches, the *primary bronchi*.

The bronchi enter the lung with blood vessels, lymphatics and nerves at a point known as the *root of the lung*.

The bronchi branch repeatedly, until the branches are very small.

These small branches are *bronchioles*.

Bronchioles eventually end at the very thin walled *alveoli* of the lungs.

Gas exchange

Red blood cells (erythrocytes) enter the lungs to rid themselves of carbon dioxide and pick up oxygen. The blood vessels keep getting smaller until they are very small capillaries in the walls of the alveoli. As the blood passes through these capillaries, the exchange of gases takes place in a split second.

Because the alveoli are very thin and cover a surface area of around 75 meters squared they provide the maximum surface area for the exchange of oxygen and carbon dioxide. This exchange or diffusion takes place through changes in pressure.

Exhalation

This is the reverse of inhalation. Air is pushed out of the lungs as the rib cage is lowered and pulled in. The diaphragm also relaxes. Exhaled air is rich in carbon dioxide, which is the main waste product from cellular respiration (energy production) in the body.

Functions

The respiratory system brings oxygen into the body, performs gas exchange in the lungs and removes waste carbon dioxide from the body.

Components

Pharynx

This is the part of the throat located behind the mouth and nasal cavity and is important in the digestive system.

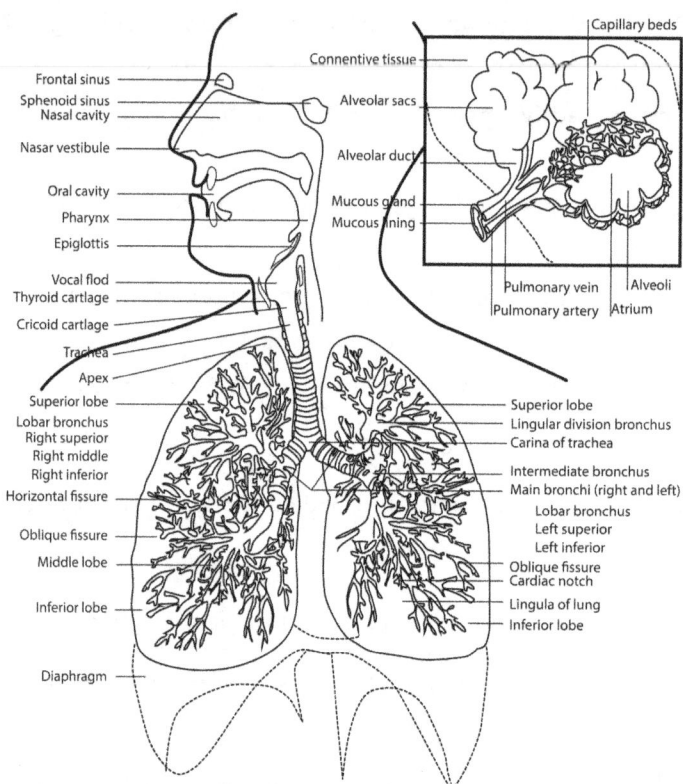

Epiglottis

This is a cartilage flap at the entrance to the voice box (larynx). When this is closed, food cannot enter the trachea (windpipe), or 'go down the wrong way'.

Larynx

The larynx or voice box allow the generation of sound with the help of varying pressures in the lungs.

Trachea

The trachea or windpipe connects the larynx to the lungs, allowing air to move between the two. It also contains goblet cells which produce mucus.

Bronchi

These passages (singular is broncus) connect the trachea to the bronchioles.

Bronchiole

Bronchioles end at the alveoli. They are typically less than 1 mm in diameter and they are able to change diameter to decrease or increase airflow.

Lungs

These are the main respiratory organs. They transport oxygen into the blood stream and release carbon dioxide. They contain many alveoli. The right lung has three lobes (sections) and the left lung is slightly smaller with two lobes, to leave room for the heart. They are composed of a variety of different tissues, including smooth muscle. The lungs of an average male can hold 6 liters of air and a woman's lungs can hold around 4 liters of air.

Rib cage

The 12 sets of ribs that make up the rib cage protect the lungs and help in the process of respiration. Between the ribs are *intercostal muscles* that move the rib cage during the respiratory cycle.

Diaphragm

This is a sheet of skeletal muscle found at the bottom of the rib cage. It separates the thoracic cavity (lungs, ribs and heart) from the abdominal cavity. The diaphragm is also essential in altering pressure in the thoracic cavity during respiration.

Alveoli

The alveoli (singular is alveolus) are the site of gas exchange in the lungs.

Common Diseases and Disorders

Asthma: The airways constrict in this chronic disease and symptoms include shortness of breath, wheezing and coughing.

Bronchitis: Infection of the bronchial tubes.

Cold/Common Cold: A cold is characterized by a sore throat, cough and runny nose. A virus from the Rhinovirus family often causes colds.

Emphysema: With exposure to heavy air pollution, often through smoking, the walls of the alveoli break down. When this occurs, the alveoli double in size and fill with fluid. Because this puts further pressure on the walls of the alveoli, they continue to break and allow fluid to accumulate. This repeats itself and destroys the lungs, impairing body function.

Flu or influenza: A virus from the influenza (Orthomyxoviridae) group of viruses causes flu. Not only is it highly infectious, flu can also cause severe illness.

Laryngitis: When people "lose their voice"; this is through infection or inflammation of the larynx. Sounds are created when air pushes by the vocal chords in the larynx. If these vocal chords are inflamed, they are unable to vibrate properly.

Pneumonia: This is infection of the lungs. Pneumonia caused by bacteria is easier to treat than infection caused by a virus. Viral pneumonia can be very serious in medically compromised people or the elderly.

Pleurisy: If the pleural cavity around the lungs becomes infected, fluid starts to accumulate. Not only does this hamper breathing, it is also very painful.

Medical Terminology

Bronchodilation: The process by which the bronchioles dilate, allowing more air to the alveoli.

Bronchoconstriction: A decrease in the diameter of bronchioles, reducing air flow.

Cilia: These are hair-like projections found on many lining cells in the body. They play an important role in moving substances along.

Coughing: This is essential to keep the lunifgs clear from debris such as mucus and dust.

Diffusion: The movement of molecules from an area of high concentration to an area of low concentration through a membrane. Diffusion allows gas exchange at the alveoli.

Mucus: Produced by certain cells, mucus often lines surfaces in the body. There are different types of mucus, but their main role is protection.

Pulmo: Any word beginning with *pulmo* relates to the lung.

Pulmonology: The branch of internal medicine that studies respiratory disorders.

Vital capacity: This is the maximum quantity of air exhaled after a maximum inspiration. This measurement is taken with a spirometer and is a frequent measure of respiratory health.

The Skeletal System

Tour of the System

The early skeleton forms during gestation and continues to develop for several years after birth through a process called endochondral ossification.

A baby has more than 300 bones, whereas an adult only has 206. This is because several bones fuse together during growth.

There are different cells involved in producing bone and these cells are located in the matrix of the bone. This matrix also contains a variety of substances and collagen. As this matrix hardens, bone forms. Formation, re-formation and repair of bones takes place over a long period of time.

Muscles, tendons, ligaments and cartilage support the skeleton and together these are the musculoskeletal system. There are several differences between male and female skeletons, including the pelvis, which has to allow for childbirth.

Functions

The skeleton has several key functions:

It supports the body and maintains the shape of the body.

The joints between the bones allow movement.

It protects organs, such as the skull protecting the brain, eyes and inner ears.

It produces cells in its bone marrow (hematopoiesis).

The skeleton stores a variety of substances including calcium and iron.

It is also involved in regulation of blood sugar levels and fat deposits through release of a hormone called oseteocalcin.

Components

Skeleton

The skeleton consists of the axial skeleton and the appendicular skeleton:

The axial skeleton is central bones including the skull, vertebrae and rib cage.

The appendicular skeleton consists of the pelvis, upper and lower limbs.

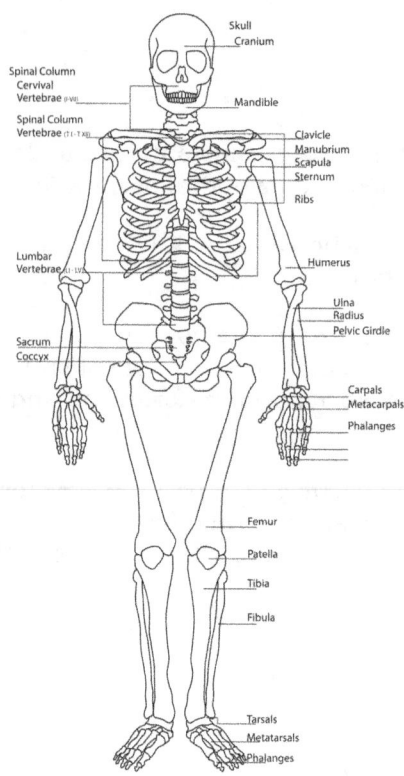

Bone

Two types of bone structure make up the skeleton:

Compact or dense bone is most of the adult skeleton. This has a smooth, white appearance.

Cancellous or *trabecular bone* is the spongy bone tissue found inside compact bone. This contains room for blood vessels and marrow.

As well as the two types of bone structure, there are also five types of bone in the human body:

Type	Description	Example
Long bones	The shaft (or diaphysis) is longer than its width	Femur, tibia, radius

Short bones	Cube shaped	Wrist bones, ankle bones
Flat bones	Thin and curved	Skull, sternum
Irregular bones	Irregular and complicated shape	Hip, spinal bones
Sesamoid bones	Found embedded in tendon	Patella (kneecap)

Joints

Joints or *articulations* are:

- where bone meets bone

- bone meets cartilage

- bone meets teeth

Joints are key components of the skeletal system. Diseases of the joints constitute the single greatest cause of disability in the civilized world.

How joints move can categorize them:

- Synarthosis: An immovable joint
- Amphiarthosis: A slightly moveable joint
- Diarthosis: Freely moveable joint

The group known as synarthoses (immovable joints) contain three joints:

1. **Suture:** This is a connective tissue joint, joining the bones of the skull. Some sutures are also present in the skeletons of children until replaced with bone. This type of temporary suture is a synostosis.

2. **Gomphosis:** A peg fits into a socket. These joints are the roots of teeth and their connection with the skull and jawbone.

3. **Synchondrosis:** This is a cartilage joint found where a bone joins to another bone with cartilage. An example is the sternocostal joints, where costal cartilage attached the ribs to the sternum (breastbone). These joints also occur in the epiphyseal (growth) plate of long bones during development. This joint eventually becomes bone.

Amphiarthoses (slightly moveable joints) contain only two sub types of joint:

1. **Syndesmosis:** Is a fibrous joint that contains more connective tissue than a suture. An example of this joint is between the tibia and fibula.

2. **Symphasis:** This joint contains a flat disc of cartilage. The main examples are the spine and hipbones.

Diarthoses or freely moveable joints (also called synovial joints) all contain a space called a synovial cavity. This cavity contains synovial fluid that lubricates and prevents friction in joints. These joints also contain cartilage that covers the ends of the bones.

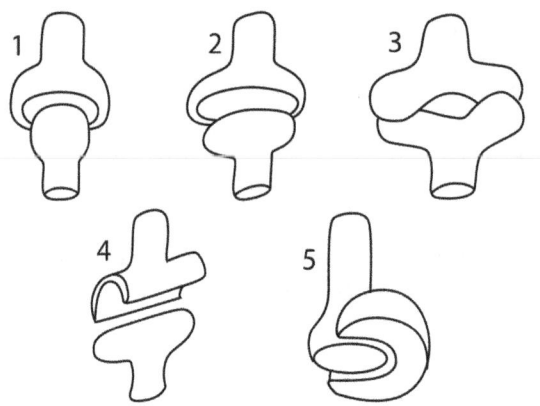

1. Ball and socket joint
2. Condyloid joint
3. Saddle joint
4. Hinge joint
5. Pivot joint

1. A ball and socket joint consists of the ball shaped end of one bone, fitting into the depression of another bone. These joints allow a variety of movement. The shoulder and hip joints are the only two ball and socket joints.
2. A condyloid joint allows side-to-side and backward and forwards movement. The joint at the wrist is a condyloid joint.
3. A saddle joint is similar to a condyloid joint, but allows more movement. The thumb is a saddle joint.
4. A hinge joint allows flexion and extension because a convex surface of one bone fits into the concave surface of another. Examples include the knee, elbow and ankle.
5. A pivot joint allows rotation of a bone. The pivot joint found at the end of the radius and ulna allows the hand to turn upwards and downwards.
6. A gliding joint allows side-to-side and backwards and forwards movement. An example is the clavicle (collarbone) gliding on the sternum (breastbone) and scapula (shoulder blade).

Muscles

Muscles help the skeleton with movement and this skeletal muscle attaches to the bones with tendons.

Tendons

Tendons are fibrous connective tissues that connect bone to muscle. These work with muscles for movement.

Ligaments

Ligaments connect bone to bone, such as the cruciate ligaments in the knee.

Cartilage

There are different types of cartilage in the body, some of which is at the joints of moveable bones, helping joints to move freely. Cartilage can also act as a shock absorber for the skeleton.

Common Diseases and Disorders

Dislocation: A dislocation or luxation occurs when bones displace at the joint. Sudden trauma, such as a fall can cause a dislocation.

Fractures: These occur when there is a break in the bone. A closed (or simple fracture) means that the skin is unbroken, whereas an open fracture has a wound at the fracture site.

Osteoporosis: This is a condition where there is a reduction in bone density, increasing the chance of fractures. This is more common in post-menopausal women, due to hormone changes.

Osteoarthritis: This is degeneration of the joints. Eventually cartilage at the end of the bones is lost

Osteomyelitis: This is infection of either the bone or its marrow.

Spur: Spurs or osteophytes form on bone as it ages, often caused with the onset of arthritis.

Medical Terminology

Collagen: This is part of connective tissue. There are many different types of collagen, found in scar tissue, skin, hair, cartilage, ligaments, bone and many other body tissues.

Connective tissue: This is a fibrous tissue with many structural roles, found in tendons, bone, cartilage and ligaments.

Endochondral ossification: Is the name for the development of the skeleton after birth.

Greenstick fracture: This fracture only occurs in children when the bones are still soft.

Haematopoiesis: The name given to the process by which different components of the blood develop in bone marrow. This includes erythrocytes, white blood cells and platelets. These all develop from stem cells.

Orthopedic: Branch of surgery concerned with the musculoskeletal system.

Strain: This occurs when a muscle is torn. It can affect also affect tendons.

Sprain: Similar to a strain, but occurs when a ligament has been over-stretched.

The Nervous System

Tour of the System

The nervous system is an incredibly complex system and along with the endocrine system, it has responsibility for maintaining homeostasis in the body. By doing this, it also controls other body systems in their functions.

The nervous system contains two main parts, the central nervous system and the peripheral nervous system:

The central nervous system (CNS) is the brain and spinal cord. This analyzes incoming sensory information, generates thoughts and emotions and creates and stores memories.

The peripheral nervous system (PNS) contains cranial nerves that come from the brain and spinal nerves that come from the spinal cord, or any other part of the nervous system that does not lie within the CNS. This can further be divided into two systems:

The sensory, or afferent (which means towards) component of the PNS takes information from nerve cells throughout the body to the CNS.

The motor, or efferent (which means away from) component of the PNS takes information from the CNS to nerve cells. There are two components to this, the somatic nervous system and the autonomic nervous system (ANS):

The somatic nervous system is voluntary. This controls information to muscles that are under voluntary control. This system is in use when we pick up a pen to start writing.

The autonomic nervous system is more complicated as it is an involuntary system. This controls information to muscles that are not under voluntary control, such as the cardiac muscle and endocrine glands. This system is controlling our heart rate, or releasing epinephrine in the body.

The key cells involved in the nervous system are nerve cells, or neurons.

Information in the nervous system is created and communicated in the form of electrical signals, created by chemical changes in neurons. These signals are nerve impulses.

This useful diagram summarizes the nervous system. The blue arrows represent information going into the nervous system (input) and the red arrows represent information going out (output) of the nervous system.

Functions

There are three main functions:

- The nervous system senses changes in the internal or external environment (changes are stimuli).

- The nervous system analyses the stimuli, stores some information about it and uses the remaining information to make decisions.

- The nervous system often responds to stimuli by starting gland secretions or muscle movements.

Components

Brain

The brain is the most complex organ in the body and not only does it control other body systems, it allows us to think, communicate and feel emotions. The brain contains mostly neurons and neuroglia cells. Tissues called meninges (inflammation of the meninges causes meningitis) and cerebrospinal fluid help to protect the brain.

Spinal cord

This extends from the *medulla oblongata* in the brain. The vertebrae of the spine protect the spinal cord. Information passes through the spinal cord to and from the brain and it is the main pathway connecting the brain and PNS.

Nerves within the spinal cord can communicate information extremely quickly and like the brain, it is protected by meninges and cerebrospinal fluid.

There are 33 nerve segments in the spine, most of which emerge from above their corresponding vertebrae:

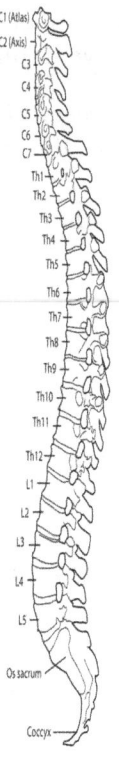

- Cervical nerve segments, identified as C1 to C8
- Thoracic nerve segments, identified as T1 to T12
- Lumbar nerve segments, identified as L1 to L5
- Sacral nerve segments, identified as S1 to S5

The spinal cord also has a special nervous response, called a reflex arc. This is when information does not enter the brain first (as there is not enough time), instead it enters the spinal cord and the spinal cord sends a message to the muscles to act.

A reflex arc occurs is when we touch something hot and we have already moved our hand away before we have 'realized' that it is hot. This response assists us in surviving.

Neurons

These vary in size from being tiny to the longest cells in the body. There are also different types of neuron, although the two main types are:

Motor neurons that communicate and control muscles.

Sensory neurons receive information from stimuli and pass this information to the CNS.

A neuron contains a cell body. This, like other cells contains the nucleus and other cell components. It also contains dendrites that extend from the cell body. These are where information (nerve impulses) enters the neuron.

The long axon allows nerve impulses to pass from the cell body to the terminal of the axon, located at the opposite end of the cell.

At the axon terminal are neurotransmitters. These molecules pass on nerve impulses to the dendrites of other neurons as well as muscles or glands.

Covering the axon is a special insulating sheath called a myelin sheath. This works like a cable covering, preventing information from being lost along the way. Breakdown of this myelin sheath causes disorders such as multiple sclerosis.

The diagram below shows how a neuron connects to its neighbors and shows where neurotransmitters are located at the axon terminals (in structures called synapses).

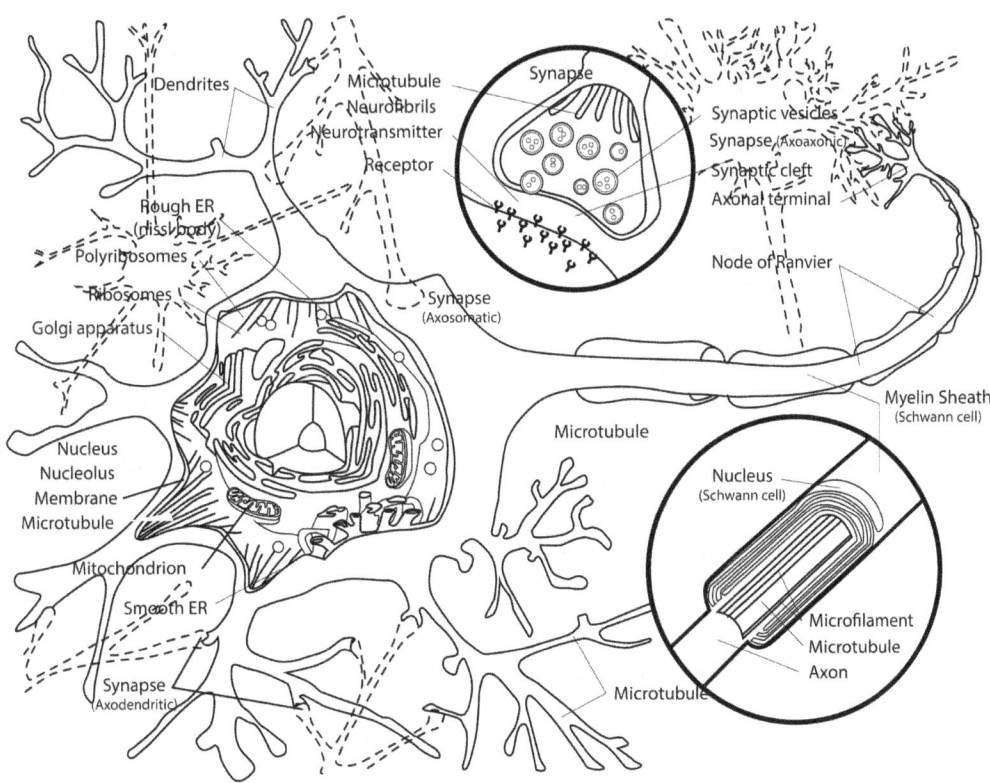

Neuroglia

Neuroglia or glia cells are not nerve cells, but they form myelin sheath for the neurons and also support and protect neurons. There are more of these than there are neurons.

Common Diseases and Disorders

Alzheimer's disease: Although the exact causes of Alzheimer's remains unknown, a breakdown of nervous tissue in the brain is involved. Neuroscientists suggest that keeping the brain active can help to delay some of the onset of Alzheimer's.

Epilepsy: Seizures are caused by abnormal electrical signals in the brain.

Multiple sclerosis (MS): This occurs with destruction of myelin sheaths of CNS neurons. This destruction prevents nerve impulses moving through the body properly.

Parkinson's disease (PD): Usually affects people around 60 years of age and causes problems with the neurotransmitters. This results in involuntary muscle movements, such as hand tremors.

Stroke: A stroke or cerebrovascular accident (CVA) occurs when blood flow to the brain is disturbed. This creates damage to the nervous tissue in the affected part of the brain. Symptoms such as slurred speech and lack of movement in one side of the body occur because of damage to the nervous tissues.

Medical Terminology

EEG (Electroencephalogram): This shows brain waves. The brain waves are the nerve impulses generated by the nervous system. These appear as electrical information.

Epidural: This is anesthetic placed in the epidural space (just inside the vertebrae) with the use of a catheter.

General anesthesia: This removes all sensations including pain and causes unconsciousness.

Homeostasis: This is the ability of the human body to maintain a stable internal environment, when dealing with both internal and external environmental changes.

Local anesthetic: Novocain and lidocaine prevents nerve impulses passing to other neurons.

Lumber puncture: Cerebrospinal fluid (CSF) is drawn from the lumber region of the spine using a needle. Often used to diagnose in disease diagnosis.

Human Body Science

Neurology: This is the branch of medicine for nervous system function and disorders.

Spinal anesthesia: This blocks nerve impulses from a certain point in the spine downwards. This is different to an epidural.

The Urinary System

Tour of the System

The urinary system removes waste by-products of metabolism. It is a very complicated system and works closely with the endocrine and cardiovascular system.

Waste products such as urea and ammonia seep from cells and tissues into the blood stream.

If these waste molecules remain in the bloodstream, they can accumulate to toxic levels in a very short time.

This liquid waste enters the kidneys through the renal arteries, from the abdominal aorta.

Around 1200 ml of blood can enter the kidneys per minute.

The renal artery entering each kidney branches into segmental arteries.

These branch into interlobar arteries.

Eventually the blood vessels become arterioles that supply the glomeruli.

The glomerulus is a ball-shaped tangled network of capillaries and is part of a nephron - the main structural and functional unit of the kidney.

Below the glomeruli is space, called the interstitium. Any fluid for re-absorption recovered from urine passes into here.

There are two main sections in the kidney, the renal cortex and renal medulla.

In the diagram below, the renal cortex is where the blood vessels are around the kidney and the renal medulla is the area between the renal pyramids.

Nephrons are located throughout the kidney and the first part of the nephron is located in the cortex. This part of the nephron, the renal corpuscle filters urine.

Nephrons have a thin wall that allows fluid to pass from the glomeruli into them.

Blood eventually drains out of nephrons into peritubular capillaries.

These then become venules and veins until filtered blood leaves the kidney through the renal vein.

Urine filtered from the blood through the nephrons passes through the renal tubule and through various tubes and processes.

It eventually reaches minor calyces and then major calyces.

The urine then enters the renal pelvis that becomes the ureter.

The ureter passes urine to the bladder.

The body makes about a liter of urine a day and this is stored in the bladder until emptying.

Urine exits the body through the urethra.

Because about one fifth of the body's supply of blood passes through the kidneys at any given time, they are terribly vulnerable to damage by toxins.

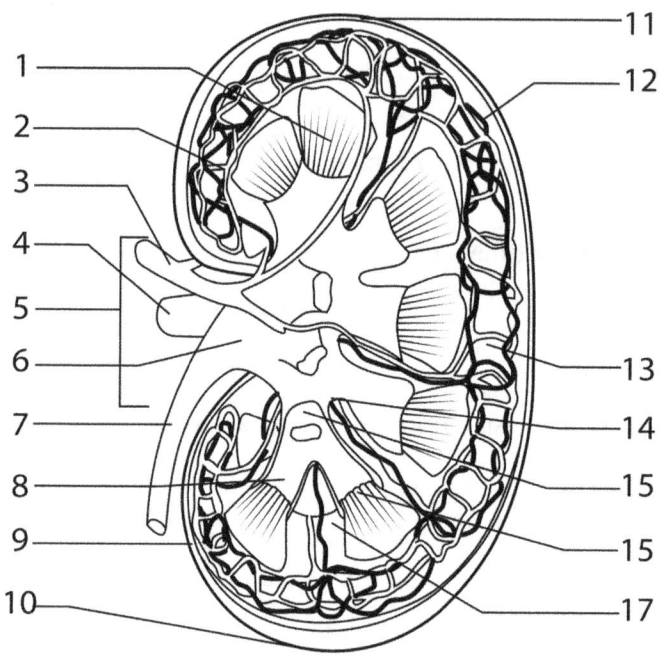

1. Renal pyramid 2. Interlobular artery 3. Renal artery 4. Renal vein 5. Renal hilum 6. Renal pelvis 7. Ureter 8. Minor calyx 9. Renal capsule 10. Inferior renal capsule 11. Superior renal capsule 12. Interlobular vein 13. Nephron 14. Minor calyx 15. Major calyx 16. Renal papilla 17. Renal column

Functions

The functions of the urinary system are to help maintain **homeostasis** by:

- Producing urine
- Storing urine
- Eliminating urine

Components

Kidneys

These are about 10-12 cm wide. As well as helping with the urinary system, kidneys also have other important functions.

They help maintain homeostasis in the body, by helping to control the composition, the volume and the pressure of blood.

Kidneys also help to control blood pH and contribute to metabolic processes such as helping the body to produce vitamin D. They also play an important role in hormone secretion.

Kidneys contain over one million nephrons and roughly 1700 liters of blood pass through these in a day. From this, 170 liters of filtrate is formed. As the filtrate passes along the nephrons, 169 liters of filtrate is reabsorbed back into the blood stream. The remaining one liter is urine.

Ureters

These two muscular tubes move urine from the kidney to the bladder. These are around 25-30 cm long and 4 mm in diameter.

Bladder

This organ collects urine from the kidneys. It is a muscular organ under both voluntary and involuntary control. As the bladder wall stretches, the nervous system contracts the detrusor muscle. This encourages urine to enter the urethra. Urine can only enter the urethra if the external sphincter, controlled voluntarily, is open.

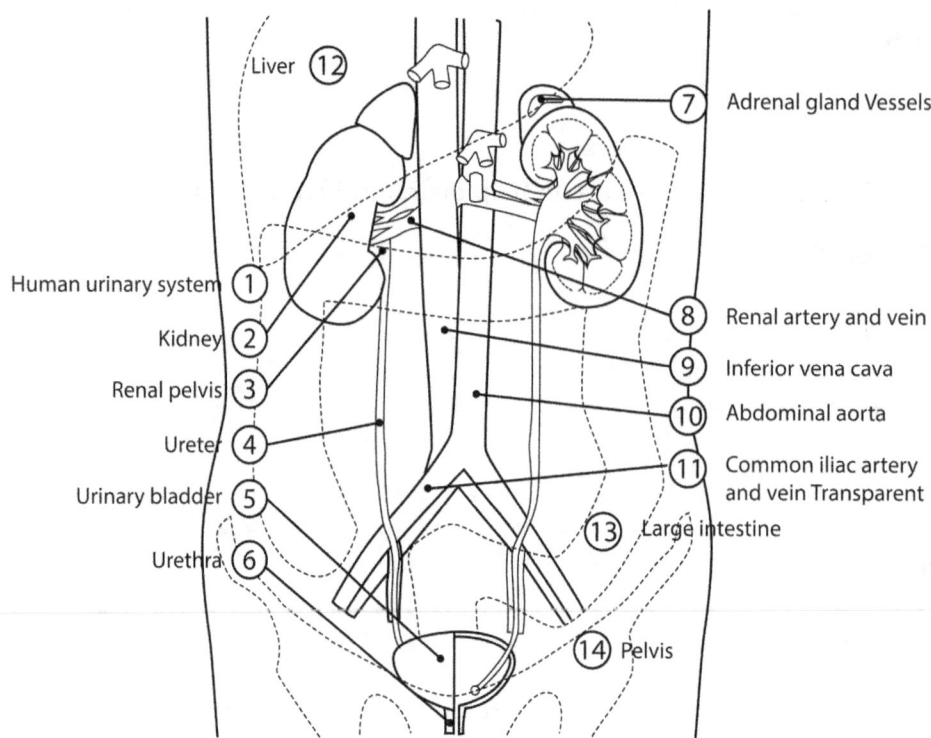

The urge to urinate usually occurs when around 25% of the bladder is full. If the bladder reaches 100% volume then the bladder will just empty. Micturition is another name for urination.

Urethra

This allows urine to exit the body. In males, the urethra also carries semen.

Testing urine can identify abnormal components that should not be in the urine, such as glucose or erythrocytes.

Common Diseases and Disorders

Acute renal failure (ARF): this is when glomerular filtration either reduces or stops. When this occurs, urine production stops. Causes include circulatory problems or kidney stones.

Chronic renal failure (CRF): This is a progressive and usually irreversible decline in filtration. This is when dialysis and a kidney transplant may be required. Kidney transplants are very successful, with the donor living with one kidney and the recipient maintaining a normal life.

Cystitis: Is a common UTI, especially in women. Cystitis is often called a bladder infection. Symptoms include a constant urge to urinate and burning when urinating.

Diabetes insipidus (DI): Is when there is a very large volume of dilute urine excreted. This is usually associated with kidney disease and is a different disorder to diabetes mellitus.

Incontinence: This usually arises from problems between voluntary and involuntary controlled muscles in the bladder.

Kidney infection: Also called pyelonephritis or pyelitis, this is a UTI that has reached the kidneys. This type of infection can be life threatening.

Kidney stones: Also known as renal calculus, these are a solid mass formed in the kidneys from minerals, such as calcium. Kidney stones can pass though the urinary system without any damage, but if they continue to grow, the ureter becomes blocked causing immense pain.

UTI or Urinary tract infection: This is any bacterial infection affecting any part of the urinary system.

Medical Terminology

Diuresis: Increased urine excretion, diuresis can be induced with diuretics, used frequently in medicine.

Homeostasis: This is the ability of the human body to maintain a stable internal environment, when dealing with both internal and external environmental changes.

Nephrology: Specialized branch of medicine dealing with the kidneys.

Polyuria: Excessive formation of urine.

Urology: Branch of medicine dealing with the urinary systems.

Immune System

Tour of the System

By taking an imaginary tour of the Immune System, we'll get a better idea of how it works and what it does.

When a virus invades the body, it first attacks a single cell. From there, the virus copies itself repeatedly until much of the body is affected--and INfected.

This is where the Immune System takes action. First, it sends a spy known as a macrophage. The macrophage figures out that the virus is an enemy and does not belong. After the tiny spy moves toward the virus, it devours it, shredding it.

The macrophage next displays antigens on its surface. Antigens are just tiny fragments of the virus. This macrophage could continue seeking out the original virus's offspring, but it would take too long. Instead, it goes for help. This help comes from a T Cell. Specifically, the macrophage finds T cells that recognize fragments from the virus on the surface of the macrophage. When the macrophage meets a T cell and the T cell recognizes traces of the virus on its surface, the T cell and macrophage physically unite.

This connecting of the cells creates a chain reaction that leads to the destruction of all copies of the virus inside the body.

How did this happen? When the T cell and macrophage connected, they released chemicals which stimulate production of more helper T cells and more macrophages. Even better, they stimulate production of a "killer" T cell.

This new killer T cell tracks down and attacks cells which are infected by the virus. Meanwhile, as the helper T cells are produced, they send out a chemical message that causes B cells to be produced. These then become plasma cells that flood the invaded body with millions of antibodies – ready to do battle.

These antibodies then track down foreign invaders, but they're more selective than the macrophages are. They are specifically seeking the strain of the virus that started the counter attack. These they flag.

The macrophages then jump in and consume these flagged viruses
If things go well, within a few days, all offspring of the virus, as well as the original virus itself, are eradicated.

Functions

The key functions of the immune system include:

- **Identifying enemies.** Specifically, immune-system cells are looking for viruses and other pathogens that have invaded healthy cells and begin reproducing, damaging the body.

- **Spotting tumors.** In the same way, the immune system is responsible for recognizing tumors in the body and beginning the process of eliminating them.

- **Destroying enemies.** Through a complex system of generating and dispatching helper cells, the immune system flags, recognizes, chases and consumes the pathogens and tumors.

- **Building future immunity.** A helpful fringe benefit is that the body develops future immunity against the virus for future attacks. This happens because of the immune system "flagging" the harmful pathogens – and allowing the immune system to recognize it in future encounters.

Components

White Blood Cells: The main soldiers in the Immune System's war against infection are white blood cells. These include:

- LEUKOCYTES. These cells act independently and are one-cell organisms that move like amoebae. Leukocytes capture pathogens by totally engulfing them.

- LYMPHOCYTES: These white blood cells travel through the person's blood looking for any foreign invader-cells. B-cell lymphocytes target bacteria with antibodies. A variety of lymphocytes known as T cells do the actual fighting.

Antibodies: Antibodies, proteins that resemble a capital "Y," respond to antigens and are produced by the white blood cells. They attach themselves to toxins and disable their signals (chemical actions). They also send out a signal to the rest of the System that this is an invader which needs to be eliminated.

Bone Marrow: The bone marrow generates new white and red blood cells. These cells then enter the blood stream, ready to do battle.
Complement System: Sometimes, germs and invaders will get through the body's natural defenses and barriers, into the blood stream. Here, liquid proteins known as complements are started and attacks the invaders. These proteins float freely within the blood stream, each reacting to a different antigen. The liver is responsible for producing complements.

Interferon: Interferon is the body's main anti-viral defense. Most of the body's cells produce interferon. Interferon's purpose is to allow the cell to send messages to other cells. This message goes something like this: I've been infected by a virus, so start producing the proteins necessary that will keep the virus outside your own structure.

Lymph Nodes: These are filters which trap foreign bodies such as germs. Working with the lymph nodes are lymphocytes, a kind of white blood cells which help the lymph nodes handle germs.

Spleen: The job of the spleen is to filter the blood as it seeks out foreign invader-cells. In addition, the spleen searches for older red cells which need to be replaced.

Thymus: Located between the heart and the breast bone, the thymus is the organ that produces T-cells that are vital for the work of the Immune System

Common Diseases and Disorders

There are three common disorders of the Immune System, described below.

Immunodeficiency are the best known, thanks largely to Human Immunodeficiency Virus (HIV, the virus that causes AIDS). An immunodeficiency occurs when certain components of the person's immune system become inactive.

Although we usually think of HIV when we think of immunodeficiency, in reality, it's common for the elderly person's immune system to start declining in their later years – a type of immunodeficiency.

Autoimmunity is the term for when the body's immune system doesn't correctly distinguish between non-self and self – and thus attacks part of the person's own body. Normally, antibodies and T cells respond with what is called "self" peptides. With autoimmunity, this process is disrupted.

Hypersensitivity is a response of the immune system which damages tissues in one's own body. There are four classes of hypersensitivity. Type 1 is an immediate reaction that we usually associate with allergy. Type 2 happens when antigens and antibodies bind together on the person's own cells, and thus marks them for destruction. Type 3 is triggered when aggregations of antigens, IgG and IgM antibodies and complements are deposited in specific tissues.

And type 4, which takes 2 or 3 days to develop, are involved in infectious diseases but can also involve skin contact (Poison Ivy is an example).. Reactions can be helped by monocytes, T cells and macrophages. [18]

Medical Terminology

Antibodies: Refers to a blood protein which is manufactured in the body as a respond to a specific antigen that has invaded the cells.
B-cells: More specifically, a B lymphocyte is one that derives from bone marrow to provide the body with humoral immunity. The B cell recognizes an antigen and transforms into plasma cells which are capable of inactivating the antigens.
Basophils: These are white blood cells that are involved with certain inflammatory reactions, especially those associated with allergies and asthma.
Bone Marrow: Found within the bones, this is fatty connective tissue that can produce the white blood cells that the immune system needs.
Complement system: This system within the immune system is made of about 30 proteins, working together to destroy infectious microorganisms. It does this by causing the bursting of foreign organisms within infected cells.
Helper T-cells: This is a T cell which recognizes antigens on the cell surface that has become infected by a virus. The helper T cell then secretes lymphokines responsible for stimulating B cells as well as killer T cells.
Interferon: A protein which is released as a response to a virus invading the body.
Killer T-cells: These are T cells that have CD8 receptors which recognize antigens on

a virus-infected cell surface.

Lymphocyte: This is a kind of white blood cell that has one single round nucleus; it occurs in a person's lymphatic system.

Macrophages: These are large phagocytic cells in tissues in stationary form or, at locations of infection, found as mobile white blood cells.

Monocytes: These are large phagocytic white cells that have simple oval nuclei plus a gray, clear cytoplasm.

Natural killer cells: These are lymphocytes which are capable of binding to virus-infected cells and tumor cells without antigens stimulating them. Once attached to the virus or tumor, they kill these invaders.

Neutrophils: These are a kind of white blood cells that are usually formed in the human bone marrow and are capable of phagocytosis.

Phagocytes: These are a kind of cell that are able to engulf and then absorb bacteria and small, harmful cells.

Plasma cells: These are B cells which manufacture one type of antibody.

Spleen: The spleen is the organ located within the abdomen that's involved in producing and removing blood cells. This vital organ is part of the immune system and is responsible for manufacturing cells that help eliminate infection, and getting rid of the infected cells.

Suppressor T-cells: The suppressor T cell suppresses or reduces an immune-system response of other T cells or of other T cells to the presence of an antigen.

T-cells: T-cells are tiny lymphocytes that are manufactured in the thymus. T-cells organize the immune system in its response to malignant or infected cells.

Thymus: The thymus is the lymphoid organ found in the neck responsible for producing many of the immune system's T-cells.

Practice Test Questions Set 1

Section I – Reading

Questions: 35
Time: 30 Minutes

Section II – Mathematics

Questions: 30
Time: 30 Minutes

Section III – English and Language Usage

Questions: 30
Time: 30 Minutes

Section IV – Science

Questions: 48
Time: 40 minutes

The questions below are not the same as you will find on the TEAS® - that would be too easy! And nobody knows what the questions will be and they change all the time. Below are general questions that cover the same subject areas as the TEAS®. While the format and exact wording of the questions may differ slightly, and change from year to year, if you can answer the questions below, you will have no problem with the TEAS®.

For the best results, take these practice test questions as if it were the real exam. Set aside time when you will not be disturbed, and a location that is quiet and free of distractions. Read the instructions carefully, read each question carefully, and answer to the best of your ability.

Use the bubble answer sheets provided. When you have completed the practice questions, check your answer against the Answer Key and read the explanation provided.

You are given 209 minutes to complete the full TEAS® exam.

Do not attempt more than one set of practice test questions in one day. After completing the first practice test, wait two or three days before attempting the second set of questions.

Section 1 - Reading

	A B C D E		A B C D E
1	○○○○○	21	○○○○○
2	○○○○○	22	○○○○○
3	○○○○○	23	○○○○○
4	○○○○○	24	○○○○○
5	○○○○○	25	○○○○○
6	○○○○○	26	○○○○○
7	○○○○○	27	○○○○○
8	○○○○○	28	○○○○○
9	○○○○○	29	○○○○○
10	○○○○○	30	○○○○○
11	○○○○○	31	○○○○○
12	○○○○○	32	○○○○○
13	○○○○○	33	○○○○○
14	○○○○○	34	○○○○○
15	○○○○○	35	○○○○○
16	○○○○○		
17	○○○○○		
18	○○○○○		
19	○○○○○		
20	○○○○○		

Section II - Math

1. A B C D 11. A B C D 21. A B C D
2. A B C D 12. A B C D 22. A B C D
3. A B C D 13. A B C D 23. A B C D
4. A B C D 14. A B C D 24. A B C D
5. A B C D 15. A B C D 25. A B C D
6. A B C D 16. A B C D 26. A B C D
7. A B C D 17. A B C D 27. A B C D
8. A B C D 18. A B C D 28. A B C D
9. A B C D 19. A B C D 29. A B C D
10. A B C D 20. A B C D 30. A B C D

Section III English

1. A B C D   11. A B C D   21. A B C D
2. A B C D   12. A B C D   22. A B C D
3. A B C D   13. A B C D   23. A B C D
4. A B C D   14. A B C D   24. A B C D
5. A B C D   15. A B C D   25. A B C D
6. A B C D   16. A B C D   26. A B C D
7. A B C D   17. A B C D   27. A B C D
8. A B C D   18. A B C D   28. A B C D
9. A B C D   19. A B C D   29. A B C D
10. A B C D   20. A B C D   30. A B C D

Section IV – Science

1. A B C D
2. A B C D
3. A B C D
4. A B C D
5. A B C D
6. A B C D
7. A B C D
8. A B C D
9. A B C D
10. A B C D
11. A B C D
12. A B C D
13. A B C D
14. A B C D
15. A B C D
16. A B C D
17. A B C D
18. A B C D
19. A B C D
20. A B C D
21. A B C D
22. A B C D
23. A B C D
24. A B C D
25. A B C D
26. A B C D
27. A B C D
28. A B C D
29. A B C D
30. A B C D
31. A B C D
32. A B C D
33. A B C D
34. A B C D
35. A B C D
36. A B C D
37. A B C D
38. A B C D
39. A B C D
40. A B C D
41. A B C D
42. A B C D
43. A B C D
44. A B C D
45. A B C D
46. A B C D
47. A B C D
48. A B C D
49. A B C D
50. A B C D

Directions: The following questions are based on several reading passages. Each passage is followed by a series of questions. Read each passage carefully, and then answer the questions based on it. You may reread the passage as often as you wish. When you have finished answering the questions based on one passage, go right onto the next passage. Choose the best answer based on the information given and implied.

Questions 1 – 4 refer to the following passage.

Passage 1 - The Life of Helen Keller

Many people have heard of Helen Keller. She is famous because she was unable to see or hear, but learned to speak and read and went onto attend college and earn a degree. Her life is a very interesting story, one that she developed into an autobiography, which was then adapted into both a stage play and a movie. How did Helen Keller overcome her disabilities to become a famous woman? Read onto find out.
Helen Keller was not born blind and deaf. When she was a small baby, she had a very high fever for several days. As a result of her sudden illness, baby Helen lost her eyesight and her hearing. Because she was so young when she went deaf and blind, Helen Keller never had any recollection of being able to see or hear. Since she could not hear, she could not learn to talk. Since she could not see, it was difficult for her to move around. For the first six years of her life, her world was very still and dark.

Imagine what Helen's childhood must have been like. She could not hear her mother's voice. She could not see the beauty of her parent's farm. She could not recognize who was giving her a hug, or a bath or even where her bedroom was each night. More sad, she could not communicate with her parents in any way. She could not express her feelings or tell them the things she wanted. It must have been a very sad childhood.

When Helen was six years old, her parents hired her a teacher named Anne Sullivan. Anne was a young woman who was almost blind. However, she could hear and she could read Braille, so she was a perfect teacher for young Helen. At first, Anne had a very hard time teaching Helen anything. She described her first impression of Helen as a "wild thing, not a child." Helen did not like Anne at first either. She bit and hit Anne when Anne tried to teach her. However, the two of them eventually came to have a great deal of love and respect.

Anne taught Helen to hear by putting her hands on people's throats. She could feel the sounds that people made. In time, Helen learned to feel what people said. Next, Anne taught Helen to read Braille, which is a way that books are written for the blind. Finally, Anne taught Helen to talk. Although Helen did learn to talk, it was hard for anyone but Anne to understand her.

As Helen grew older, more and more people were amazed by her story. She went to college and wrote books about her life. She gave talks to the public, with Anne at her side, translating her words. Today, both Anne Sullivan and Helen Keller are famous women who are respected for their lives' work.

1. Helen Keller could not see and hear and so, what was her biggest problem in childhood?

    a. Inability to communicate

    b. Inability to walk

    c. Inability to play

    d. Inability to eat

2. Helen learned to hear by feeling the vibrations people made when they spoke. What were these vibrations were felt through?

    a. Mouth

    b. Throat

    c. Ears

    d. Lips

3. From the passage, we can infer that Anne Sullivan was a patient teacher. We can infer this because

    a. Helen hit and bit her and Anne still remained her teacher.

    b. Anne taught Helen to read only.

    c. Anne was hard of hearing too.

    d. Anne wanted to be a teacher.

4. Helen Keller learned to speak but Anne translated her words when she spoke in public. The reason Helen needed a translator was because

    a. Helen spoke another language.

    b. Helen's words were hard for people to understand.

    c. Helen spoke very quietly.

    d. Helen did not speak but only used sign language.

Questions 5 – 8 refer to the following passage.

Passage 2 - Ways Characters Communicate in Theater

Playwrights give their characters voices in a way that gives depth and added meaning to what happens on stage during their play. There are different types of speech in scripts that allow characters to talk with themselves, with other characters, and even with the audience.

It is very unique to theater that characters may talk "to themselves." When characters do this, the speech they give is called a soliloquy. Soliloquies are usually poetic, introspective, moving, and can tell audience members about the feelings, motivations, or suspicions of an individual character without that character having to reveal them to other characters on stage. "To be or not to be" is a famous soliloquy given by Hamlet as he considers difficult but important themes, such as life and death.

The most common type of communication in plays is when one character is speaking to another or a group of other characters. This is generally called dialogue, but can also be called monologue if one character speaks without being interrupted for a long time. It is not necessarily the most important type of communication, but it is the most common because the plot of the play cannot really progress without it.

Lastly, and most unique to theater (although it has been used somewhat in film) is when a character speaks directly to the audience. This is called an aside, and scripts usually specifically direct actors to do this. Asides are usually comical, an inside joke between the character and the audience, and very short. The actor will usually face the audience when delivering them, even if it's for a moment, so the audience can recognize this move as an aside.

All three of these types of communication are important to the art of theater, and have been perfected by famous playwrights like Shakespeare. Understanding these types of communication can help an audience member grasp what is artful about the script and action of a play.

5. According to the passage, characters in plays communicate to

    a. move the plot forward

    b. show the private thoughts and feelings of one character

    c. make the audience laugh

    d. add beauty and artistry to the play

6. When Hamlet delivers "To be or not to be," he can most likely be described as

    a. solitary

    b. thoughtful

    c. dramatic

    d. hopeless

7. The author uses parentheses to punctuate "although it has been used somewhat in film,"

    a. to show that films are less important

    b. instead of using commas so that the sentence is not interrupted

    c. because parenthesis help separate details that are not as important

    d. to show that films are not as artistic

Questions 9 – 11 refer to the following passage.

Passage 3 - Low Blood Sugar

As the name suggest, low blood sugar is low sugar levels in the bloodstream. This can occur when you have not eaten properly and undertake strenuous activity, or, when you are very hungry. When Low blood sugar occurs regularly and is ongoing, it is a medical condition called hypoglycemia. This condition can occur in diabetics and in healthy adults.

Causes of low blood sugar can include excessive alcohol consumption, metabolic problems, stomach surgery, pancreas, liver or kidneys problems, as well as a side-effect of some medications.

Symptoms

There are different symptoms depending on the severity of the case.

Mild hypoglycemia can lead to feelings of nausea and hunger. The patient may also feel nervous, jittery and have fast heart beats. Sweaty skin, clammy and cold skin are likely symptoms.
Moderate hypoglycemia can result in a short temper, confusion, nervousness, fear and blurring of vision. The patient may feel weak and unsteady.

Severe cases of hypoglycemia can lead to seizures, coma, fainting spells, nightmares, headaches, excessive sweats and severe tiredness.

Diagnosis of low blood sugar

A doctor can diagnosis this medical condition by asking the patient questions and testing blood and urine samples. Home testing kits are available for patients to monitor blood sugar levels. It is important to see a qualified doctor though. The doctor can administer tests to ensure that will safely rule out other medical conditions that could affect blood sugar levels.

Treatment

Quick treatments include drinking or eating foods and drinks with high sugar contents. Good examples include soda, fruit juice, hard candy and raisins. Glucose energy tablets can also help. Doctors may also recommend medications and well as changes in diet and exercise routine to treat chronic low blood sugar.

8. Based on the article, which of the following is true?

    a. Low blood sugar can happen to anyone.

    b. Low blood sugar only happens to diabetics.

    c. Low blood sugar can occur even.

    d. None of the statements are true.

Practice Test Questions Set 1

9. Which of the following are the author's opinion?

a. Quick treatments include drinking or eating foods and drinks with high sugar contents.

b. None of the statements are opinions.

c. This condition can occur in diabetics and also in healthy adults.

d. There are different symptoms depending on the severity of the case

10. What is the author's purpose?

a. To inform

b. To persuade

c. To entertain

d. To analyze

11. Which of the following is not a detail?

a. A doctor can diagnosis this medical condition by asking the patient questions and testing.

b. A doctor will test blood and urine samples.

c. Glucose energy tablets can also help.

d. Home test kits monitor blood sugar levels.

Questions 12 – 14 refer to the following passage.

How To Get A Good Nights Sleep

Sleep is just as essential for healthy living as water, air and food. Sleep allows the body to rest and replenish depleted energy levels. Sometimes we may for various reasons experience difficulty sleeping which has a serious effect on our
health. Those who have prolonged sleeping problems are facing a serious medical condition and should see a qualified doctor when possible for help. Here is simple guide that can help you sleep better at night.

Try to create a natural pattern of waking up and sleeping around the same time everyday. This means avoiding going to bed too early and oversleeping past your usual wake up time. Going to bed and getting up at radically different times everyday confuses your body clock. Try to establish a natural rhythm as much as you can.

Exercises and a bit of physical activity can help you sleep better at night. If you are having problem sleeping, try to be as active as you can during the day. If you are tired from physical activity, falling asleep is a natural and easy process
for your body. If you remain inactive during the day, you will find it harder to sleep

properly at night. Try walking, jogging, swimming or simple stretches as you get close to your bed time.

Afternoon naps are great to refresh you during the day, but they may also keep you awake at night. If you feel sleepy during the day, get up, take a walk and get busy to keep from sleeping. Stretching is a good way to increase blood flow to the brain and keep you alert so that you don't sleep during the day. This will help you sleep better night.

A warm bath or a glass of milk in the evening can help your body relax and prepare for sleep. A cold bath will wake you up and keep you up for several hours. Also avoid eating too late before bed.

12. How would you describe this sentence?

    a. A recommendation

    b. An opinion

    c. A fact

    d. A diagnosis

13. Which of the following is an alternative title for this article?

    a. Exercise and a good night's sleep

    b. Benefits of a good night's sleep

    c. Tips for a good night's sleep

    d. Lack of sleep is a serious medical condition

14. Which of the following cannot be inferred from this article?

    a. Biking is helpful for getting a good night's sleep

    b. Mental activity is helpful for getting a good night's sleep

    c. Eating bedtime snacks is not recommended

    d. Getting up at the same time is helpful for a good night's sleep

15. What is a disadvantage of taking naps?

    a. They may keep you awake.

    b. There are no disadvantages

    c. They may help you sleep better

    d. They may affect your diet

Question 16 refers to the following Table of Contents.

Contents

Contents

    Science Self-assessment 81
    Answer Key 91
    Science Tutorials 96
    Scientific Method 96
    Biology 99
    Heredity: Genes and Mutation 104
    Classification 108
    Ecology 110
    Chemistry 112
    Energy: Kinetic and Mechanical 126
    Energy: Work and Power 130
    Force: Newton's Three Laws 132

16. Consider the table of contents above. What page would you find information about natural selection and adaptation?

    a. 81

    b. 90

    c. 110

    d. 132

Questions 17 – 19 refer to the following passage.

Passage 5 - Pearl Harbor

A Day That Will Live in Infamy! Attack on Pearl Harbor
In 1941, the world was at war. The United States was trying very hard to keep itself out of the conflict. In Europe, the countries of Germany and Italy had formed an alliance to expand their land and territory. Germany had already taken over Poland, Denmark, and parts of France. They were heading next toward England and due to all the fighting in Europe, there were battles taking place as far south as North Africa, where the German

and Italian armies were fighting the British.

This got even worse when the Asian nation of Japan formed an alliance with Germany and Italy. Together, the three countries called themselves, the AXIS. Now, the war was in the Pacific as well as in Europe and Northern Africa. A great deal of Americans felt that perhaps now was the time for the United States to join with its ally, Great Britain and stop the Axis from taking over more regions of the world.

In 1941, Franklin Roosevelt was President of the United States. His fear at the time was that Japan would try to take over many countries in Asia. He did not want to see that happen, so he moved some of the United States warships that had been stationed in San Diego, to the military base at Pearl Harbor, in Honolulu, Hawaii.

Japan quietly plotted their attack. They waited until the early hours of the morning on Sunday, December 7, 1941. Then, 350 Japanese war plans began to drop bombs on the U.S. ships at Pearl Harbor. The first bombs fell at 7:48 am and a mere 90 minutes later, the attack was over. Pearl Harbor was decimated. 8 battleships were damaged. Eleven ships were sunk and 300 U.S. planes were destroyed. Most devastating was the loss of life 2,400 U.S. military members was killed in the attack and 1,282 were injured.

President Roosevelt addressed the country via the radio and said "Today is a day that will live in infamy." He asked Congress to declare war on Japan. War was declared on Japan on December 8th and on Germany and Italy on December 11th. The United States had entered World War Two.

17. After reading the passage, what can you infer infamy means?

    a. Famous

    b. Remembered in a good way

    c. Remembered in a bad way

    d. Easily forgotten

18. What three countries formed the Axis?

    a. Italy, England, Germany

    b. United States, England, Italy

    c. Germany, Japan, Italy

    d. Germany, Japan, United States

19. What do you think was President Roosevelt's reason for moving warships to Pearl Harbor?

    a. He feared Japan would bomb San Diego

    b. He knew Japan was going to attack Pearl Harbor

    c. He was planning to attack Japan

    d. He wanted to try and protect Asian countries from Japanese takeover

20. Why do you think Japan chose a Sunday morning at 7:48 am for their attack?

    a. They knew the military slept late

    b. There is a law against bombing countries on a Sunday

    c. They wanted the attack to catch people by surprise

    d. That was the only free time they had to attack.

Questions 21 - 24 refer to the following recipe.

If You Have Allergies, You're Not Alone

People who experience allergies might joke that their immune systems have let them down or are seriously lacking. Truthfully though, people who experience allergic reactions or allergy symptoms during certain times of the year have heightened immune systems that are, "better" than those of people who have perfectly healthy but less militant immune systems.

Still, when a person has an allergic reaction, they are having an adverse reaction to a substance that is considered normal to most people. Mild allergic reactions usually have symptoms like itching, runny nose, red eyes, or bumps or discoloration of the skin. More serious allergic reactions, such as those to animal and insect poisons or certain foods, may result in the closing of the throat, swelling of the eyes, low blood pressure, inability to breath, and can even be fatal.

Different treatments help different allergies, and which one a person uses depends on the nature and severity of the allergy. It is recommended to patients with severe allergies to take extra precautions, such as carrying an EpiPen, which treats anaphylactic shock and may prevent death, always in order for the remedy to be readily available and more effective. When an allergy is not so severe, treatments may be used just relieve a person of uncomfortable symptoms. Over the counter allergy medicines treat milder symptoms, and can be bought at any grocery store and used in moderation to help people with allergies live normally.

There are many tests available to assess whether a person has allergies or what they may be allergic to, and advances in these tests and the medicine used to treat patients continues to improve. Despite this fact, allergies still affect many people throughout the year or even every day. Medicines used to treat allergies have side effects of their own, and it is difficult to bring the body into balance with the use of medicine. Regardless, many of those who live with allergies are grateful for what is available and find it useful in maintaining their lifestyles.

21. According to this passage, it can be understood that the word "militant" belongs in a group with the words:

   a. sickly, ailing, faint

   b. strength, power, vigor

   c. active, fighting, warring

   d. worn, tired, breaking down

22. The author says that "medicines used to treat allergies have side-effects of their own" to

   a. point out that doctors aren't very good at diagnosing and treating allergies

   b. argue that because of the large number of people with allergies, a cure will never be found

   c. explain that allergy medicines aren't cures and some compromise must be made

   d. argue that more wholesome remedies should be researched and medicines banned

23. It can be inferred that _____ recommend that some people with allergies carry medicine with them.

   a. the author

   b. doctors

   c. the makers of EpiPen

   d. people with allergies

24. The author has written this passage to

   a. inform readers on symptoms of allergies so people with allergies can get help

   b. persuade readers to be proud of having allergies

   c. inform readers on different remedies so people with allergies receive the right help

   d. describe different types of allergies, their symptoms, and their remedies

Questions 25 – 26 refer to the following email.

SUBJECT: MEDICAL STAFF CHANGES

To all staff:

This email is to advise you of a paper on recommended medical staff changes has been posted to the Human Resources website.

The contents are of primary interest to medical staff, other staff may be interested in reading it, particularly those in medical support roles.

The paper deals with several major issues:

1. Improving our ability to attract top quality staff to the hospital, and retain our existing staff. These changes will make our position and departmental names internationally recognizable and comparable with North American and North Asian departments and positions.

2. Improving our ability to attract top quality staff by introducing greater flexibility in the departmental structure.

3. General comments on issues to be further discussed in relation to research staff.

The changes outlined in this paper are significant. I encourage you to read the document and send to me any comments you may have, so that it can be enhanced and improved.

Gordon Simms
Administrator,
Seven Oaks Regional Hospital

25. Are all hospital staff required to read the document posted to the Human Resources website?

    a. Yes all staff are required to read the document.

    b. No, reading the document is optional.

    c. Only medical staff are required to read the document.

    d. none of the above are correct.

26. Have the changes to medical staff been made?

    a. Yes, the changes have been made.

    b. No, the changes are only being discussed.

    c. Some of the changes have been made.

    d. None of the choices are correct.

Questions 27 – 30 refer to the following passage.

When a Poet Longs to Mourn, He Writes an Elegy

Poems are an expressive, especially emotional, form of writing. They have been present in literature virtually from the time civilizations invented the written word. Poets often portrayed as moody, secluded, and even troubled, but this is because poets are introspective and feel deeply about the current events and cultural norms they are surrounded with. Poets often produce the most telling literature, giving insight into the society and mind-set they come from. This can be done in many forms.

The oldest types of poems often include many stanzas, may or may not rhyme, and are more about telling a story than experimenting with language or words. The most common types of ancient poetry are epics, which are usually extremely long stories that follow a hero through his journey, or ellegies, which are often solemn in tone and used to mourn or lament something or someone. The Mesopotamians are often said to have invented the written word, and their literature is among the oldest in the world, including the epic poem titled "Epic of Gilgamesh." Similar in style and length to "Gilgamesh" is "Beowulf," an ellegy written in Old English and set in Scandinavia. These poems are often used by professors as the earliest examples of literature.

The importance of poetry was revived in the Renaissance. At this time, Europeans discovered the style and beauty of ancient Greek arts, and poetry was among those. Shakespeare is the most well-known poet of the time, and he used poetry not only to write poems but also to write plays for the theater. The most popular forms of poetry during the Renaissance included villanelles, (a nineteen-line poetic form) sonnets, as well as the epic. Poets during this time focused on style and form, and developed very specific rules and outlines for how an exceptional poem should be written.

As often happens in the arts, modern poets have rejected the constricting rules of Renaissance poets, and free form poems are much more popular. Some modern poems would read just like stories if they weren't arranged into lines and stanzas. It is difficult to tell which poems and poets will be the most important, because works of art often become more famous in hindsight, after the poet has died and society can look at itself without being in the moment. Modern poetry continues to develop, and will no doubt continue to change as values, thought, and writing continue to change.

Poems can be among the most enlightening and uplifting texts for a person to read if they are looking to connect with the past, connect with other people, or try to gain an understanding of what is happening in their time.

27. In summary, the author has written this passage

    a. as a foreword that will introduce a poem in a book or magazine

    b. because she loves poetry and wants more people to like it

    c. to give a brief history of poems

    d. to convince students to write poems

28. The author organizes the paragraphs mainly by

a. moving chronologically, explaining which types of poetry were common in that time

b. talking about new types of poems each paragraph and explaining them a little

c. focusing on one poet or group of people and the poems they wrote

d. explaining older types of poetry so she can talk about modern poetry

29. The author's claim that poetry has been around "virtually from the time civilizations invented the written word" is supported by the detail that

a. Beowulf is written in Old English, which is not really in use any longer

b. epic poems told stories about heroes

c. the Renaissance poets tried to copy Greek poets

d. the Mesopotamians are credited with both inventing the word and writing "Epic of Gilgamesh"

30. According to the passage, it can be understood that the word "telling" means

a. speaking

b. significant

c. soothing

d. wordy

Questions 31 – 32 refer to the following passage.

Scottish Wind Farms

The Scottish Government has a targeted plan of generating 100% of Scotland's electricity through renewable energy by 2020. Renewable energy sources include sun, water and wind power. Scotland uses all forms but its fastest growing energy is wind energy. Wind power is generated through the use of wind turbines, placed onshore and offshore. Wind turbines that are grouped together in large numbers are called wind farms. A majority of Scottish citizens say that the wind farms are necessary to meet current and future energy needs, and would like to see an increase in the number of wind farms. They cite the fact that wind energy does not cause pollution, there are low operational costs, and most importantly due to the definition of renewable energy it cannot be depleted.

31. What is Scotland's fastest growing source of renewable energy?

a. Solar Panels
b. Hydroelectric
c. Wind
d. Fossil Fuels

32. Why do the majority of Scottish citizens agree with the Government's plan?

a. Their concern for current and future energy needs
b. Because of the low operational costs
c. Because they are out of sight
d. Because it provides jobs

Questions 33 – 34 refer to the following passage.

Scottish Wind Farms II

However, there is still a public debate concerning the use of wind farms to generate energy. The most cited argument against wind energy is that the upfront investment is expensive. They also argue that it is aesthetically displeasing, they are noisy, and they create a serious threat to wildlife in the area. While wind energy is renewable, or cannot be depleted, it does not mean that wind is always available. Wind is fluctuating, or intermittent, and therefore not suited to meet the base amount of energy demand, meaning if there is no wind then no energy is being created.

33. What is the biggest argument against wind energy?

a. The turbines are noisy
b. The turbines endanger wildlife
c. The turbines are expensive to build
d. They are aesthetically displeasing

34. What is the best way to describe this article's description of wind energy?

a. Loud and ever present
b. The cheapest form of renewable energy
c. The only source of renewable energy in Scotland
d. Clean and renewable but fluctuating

Save the Children

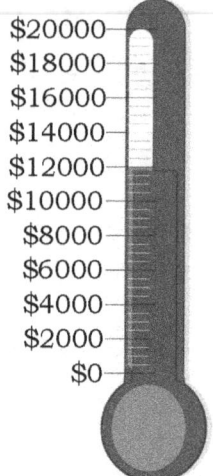

35. Consider the graphic above. The Save the Children fund has a fund-raising goal of $20,000. Approximately how much of their goal have they achieved?

a. 3/5
b. 3/4
c. 1/2
d. 1/3

Section II – Math

1. What is 1/3 of 3/4?

  a. 1/4
  b. 1/3
  c. 2/3
  d. 3/4

2. Susan wants to buy a leather jacket that costs $545.00 and is on sale for 10% off. What is the approximate cost?

  a. $525
  b. $450
  c. $475
  d. $500

3. 3.14 + 2.73 + 23.7 =

  a. 28.57
  b. 30.57
  c. 29.56
  d. 29.57

4. A woman spent 15% of her income on an item and ends with $120. What percentage of her income is left?

  a. 12%
  b. 85%
  c. 75%
  d. 95%

5. Express 0.27 + 0.33 as a fraction.

  a. 3/6
  b. 4/7
  c. 3/5
  d. 2/7

6. 8 is what percent of 40?

  a. 10%
  b. 15%
  c. 20%
  d. 25%

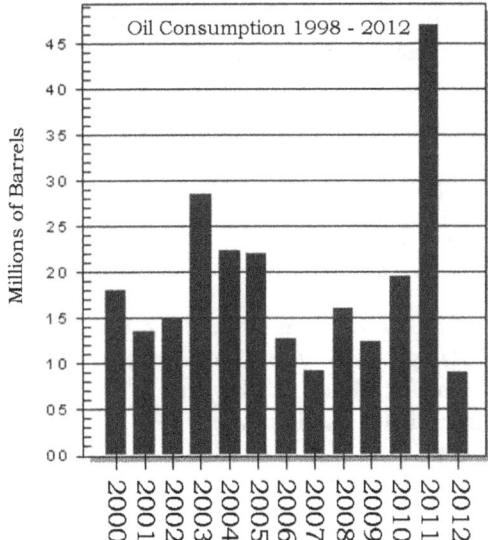

7. The graph above shows oil consumption in millions of barrels for the period, 1998 - 2012. What year did oil consumption peak?

  a. 2011
  b. 2010
  c. 2008
  d. 2009

8. Translate the following into an equation: 2 + a number divided by 7.

  a. (2 + X)/7
  b. (7 + X)/2
  c. (2 + 7)/X
  d. 2/(7 + X)

9. .4% of 36 is

   a. 1.44
   b. .144
   c. 14.4
   d. 144

10. The physician ordered 5 mg Coumadin; 10 mg/tablet is on hand. How many tablets will you give?

    a. .5 tablet
    b. 1 tablet
    c. .75 tablet
    d. 1.5 tablets

11. The physician ordered 20 mg Tylenol/kg of body weight; on hand is 80 mg/tablet. The child weighs 12 kg. How many tablets will you give?

    a. 1 tablet
    b. 3 tablets
    c. 2 tablets
    d. 4 tablets

12. Consider the following population growth chart.

Country	Population 2000	Population 2005
Japan	122,251,000	128,057,000
China	1,145,195,000	1,341,335,000
United States	253,339,000	310,384,000
Indonesia	184,346,000	239,871,000

What country is growing the fastest?

   a. Japan
   b. China
   c. United States
   d. Indonesia

13. If y = 4 and x = 3, solve yx^3

    a. -108
    b. 108
    c. 27
    d. 4

14. What number is MCMXC?

    a. 1990
    b. 1980
    c. 2000
    d. 1995

15. Convert 16 quarts to gallons.

    a. 1 gallons
    b. 8 gallons
    c. 4 gallons
    d. 4.5 gallons

16. Convert 45 kg. to pounds.

    a. 10 pounds
    b. 100 pounds
    c. 1,000 pounds
    d. 110 pounds

17. Translate the following into an equation: three plus a number times 7 equals 42.

   a. 7(3 + X) = 42
   b. 3(X + 7) = 42
   c. 3X + 7 = 42
   d. (3 + 7)X = 42

18. In a class of 83 students, 72 are present. What percent of the students are absent? Provide answer up to two significant digits.

   a. 12%
   b. 13%
   c. 14%
   d. 15%

19. 5x+2(x+7) = 14x – 7. Find x

   a. 1
   b. 2
   c. 3
   d. 4

20. 5(z+1) = 3(z+2) + 11. Find z

   a. 2
   b. 4
   c. 6
   d. 12

21. The price of a book went from $20 to $25. What percent did the price increase?

   a. 5%
   b. 10%
   c. 20%
   d. 25%

22. A boy is given 2 apples while his sister is given 8 oranges. What is the ratio between the boy's apples and her oranges?

   a. 1:2
   b. 2:4
   c. 1:4
   d. 2:1

23. In the time required to serve 43 customers, a server breaks 2 glasses and slips 5 times. The next day, the same server breaks 10 glasses. Assuming that glasses broken is proportional to customers served, how many customers did she serve?

   a. 25
   b. 43
   c. 86
   d. 215

24. A square lawn has an area of 62,500 square meters. What is the cost of building fence around it at a rate of $5.5 per meter?

   a. $4000
   b. $4500
   c. $5000
   d. $5500

25. Solve for n, when 5n + (19 – 2) = 67.

   a. 21
   b. 10
   c. 15
   d. 7

26. Below is the attendance for a class of 45.

Day	Absent Students
Monday	5
Tuesday	9
Wednesday	4
Thursday	10
Friday	6

What is the average attendance for the week?

   a. 88%
   b. 85%
   c. 81%
   d. 77%

27. A distributor purchased 550 kilograms of potatoes for $165. He distributed these at a rate of $6.4 per 20 kilograms to 15 shops, $3.4 per 10 kilograms to 12 shops and the remainder at $1.8 per 5 kilograms. If his total distribution cost is $10, what will his profit be?

   a. $10.40
   b. $8.60
   c. $14.90
   d. $23.40

28. How much pay does Mr. Johnson receive if he gives half of his pay to his family, $250 to his landlord, and has exactly 3/7 of his pay left over?

   a. $3600
   b. $3500
   c. $2800
   d. $1750

29. A boy has 4 red, 5 green and 2 yellow balls. He chooses two balls randomly. What is the probability that one is red and other is green?

   a. 2/11
   b. 19/22
   c. 20/121
   d. 9/11

30. The cost of waterproofing canvas is .50 a square yard. What's the total cost for waterproofing a canvas truck cover that is 15' x 24'?

   a. $18.00
   b. $6.67
   c. $180.00
   d. $20.00

Section III - English

1. Choose the sentence with the correct grammar.

   a. Don would never have thought of that book, but you could have reminded him.

   b. Don would never of thought of that book, but you could have reminded him.

   c. Don would never have thought of that book, but you could of have reminded him.

   d. Don would never of thought of that book, but you could of reminded him.

2. Choose the correct sentence.

   a. The boy and girl are related.

   b. The boy and girl is related.

   c. The boy and girl was related.

   d. None of the above.

3. Choose the sentence with the correct grammar.

   a. There was scarcely no food in the pantry, because nobody ate at home.

   b. There was scarcely any food in the pantry, because nobody ate at home.

   c. There was scarcely any food in the pantry, because not nobody ate at home.

   d. There was scarcely no food in the pantry, because not nobody ate at home.

4. Choose the sentence with the correct grammar.

   a. Its important for you to know its official name; its called the Confederate Museum.

   b. It's important for you to know it's official name; it's called the Confederate Museum.

   c. It's important for you to know its official name; it's called the Confederate Museum.

   d. Its important for you to know it's official name; it's called the Confederate Museum.

5. Choose the sentence with the correct grammar.

   a. The man as well as his son has arrived.

   b. The man as well as his son have arrived.

   c. Both of the above.

   d. None of the above.

6. Thomas Edison _____ since he invented the light bulb, television, motion pictures, and phonograph.

   a. has always been known as the greatest inventor
   b. was always been known as the greatest inventor
   c. must have had been always known as the greatest inventor
   d. will had been known as the greatest inventor

7. The weatherman on Channel 6 said that this has been the

   a. most hottest summer on record
   b. most hotter summer on record
   c. hottest summer on record
   d. hotter summer on record

8. Although Joe is tall for his age, his brother Elliot is _____ of the two.

   a. the tallest
   b. more tallest
   c. the tall
   d. the taller

9. When KISS came to town, all of the tickets _____ before I could buy one.

   a. will be sold out
   b. had been sold out
   c. were being sold out
   d. was sold out

10. The rules of most sports _____ more complicated than we often realize.

    a. are
    b. is
    c. was
    d. has been

11. _____ won first place in the Western Division?

    a. Who
    b. Whom
    c. Which
    d. What

Practice Test Questions Set 1

12. There are now several ways to listen to music, including radio, CDs, and Mp3 files _____ you can download onto an MP3 player.

    a. on which
    b. who
    c. whom
    d. which

13. Choose the sentence with the correct grammar.

    a. Each of them have to be given a ticket.
    b. Each of them is to be given a ticket.
    c. Each of them are to be given a ticket.
    d. None of the above.

14. Choose the correct spelling.

    a. maintainance
    b. maintenace
    c. maintanance
    d. maintenance

15. Choose the correct spelling.

    a. humoros
    b. humouros
    c. humorous
    d. humorus

16. Choose the correct spelling.

    a. mathematics
    b. mathmatics
    c. matematics
    d. mathamatics

17. Choose the sentence below with the correct punctuation.

a. Ted and Janice, who had been friends for years, went on vacation together every summer.

b. Ted and Janice, who had been friends for years, went on vacation together, every summer.

c. Ted, and Janice who had been friends for years, went on vacation together every summer.

d. Ted and Janice who had been friends for years went on vacation together every summer.

18. Choose the sentence with the correct capitalization.

a. The Sahara Desert is found in the northern part of Africa.

b. The Sahara Desert is found in the Northern part of Africa.

c. The Sahara desert is found in the northern part of Africa.

d. The Sahara desert is found in the Northern part of Africa.

19. She went with him to the dance.

What is the subject of this sentence?

a. She
b. Dance
c. Him
d. With

20. She studied long and hard and her marks showed it.

What is the predicate of this sentence?

a. Studied long and hard
b. Marks showed it
c. Showed it
d. None of the above

Practice Test Questions Set 1

21. What is on the test?

What type of sentence is this?

    a. Imperative
    b. Interrogative
    c. Exclamatory
    d. Declarative

22. The aquarium featured brightly-colored tropical fish that came from the tropics.

What part of this sentence is redundant?

    a. Brightly-colored
    b. Tropical fish
    c. That came from the tropics
    d. Aquarium

23. Choose the correct sentence.

    a. Historians have been guessing the doctor was a woman for more than 100 years.
    b. Historians have been guessing for more than 100 years the doctor was a woman.
    c. Historians guessed the doctor was a woman for more than 100 years.
    d. None of the above.

24. Choose the correct sentence.

    a. None of us want to go to the party not even, if there will be live music.
    b. None of us want to go to the party, not even if there will be live music.
    c. None of us want to go to the party not even if there will be live music.
    d. None of us want to go to the party; not even if there will be live music.

25. Choose the correct sentence.

    a. I own two dogs, a cat named Jeffrey, and Henry, the goldfish.
    b. I own two dogs a cat, named Jeffrey, and Henry, the goldfish.
    c. I own two dogs, a cat named Jeffrey; and Henry, the goldfish.
    d. I own two dogs, a cat, named Jeffrey and Henry, the goldfish.

26. Choose the correct sentence.

   a. During the years he was President, the country fought two wars.
   b. During the years he was president, the country fought two wars.
   c. During the years he was president, the Country fought two wars.
   d. During the years he was President, the Country fought two wars.

27. Alice <u>jumped</u> when she saw the rabbit.

What part of speech is the underlined word?

   a. Noun
   b. Verb
   c. Adjective
   d. Adverb

28. Which of the following sentences contains a redundant phrase?

   a. I will be leaving shortly.
   b. I think the situation calls for a direct confrontation.
   c. The fish swam upstream with great difficulty.
   d. None of the above.

Directions: For each of the questions below, choose the word with the meaning best suited to the sentence based on the context.

29. Paul's rose bushes were being destroyed by Japanese beetles, so he invested in a good _____.

   a. Fungicide
   b. Fertilizer
   c. Sprinkler
   d. Pesticide

30. Because of a pituitary dysfunction, Karl lacked the necessary _____ to grow as tall as his father.

   a. Glands
   b. Hormones
   c. Vitamins
   d. Testosterone

Section III – Science

1. Describe the differences between genotypes and phenotypes.

a. Phenotype refers to observed properties of an organism and genotype refers to the genes of an organism.

b. Genotype refers to observed properties of an organism and phenotype refers to the genes of an organism.

c. Phenotype refers to the DNA of an organism and genotype refers to the genes of an organism.

d. Genotype refers to the DNA of an organism and phenotype refers to the genes of an organism.

2. A solution with a pH value of greater than 7 is

a. Base.
b. Acid.
c. Neutral.
d. None of the above.

3. Which statement below regarding Eukaryotic and prokaryotic cells is correct?

a. Both are organelles
b. Eukaryotic are not organelles
c. Both have DNA
d. Both have single membrane compartments

4. When we say that important traits for scientific classification are homologous, "homologous" means

a. Being shared among two or more animals with the same parent.
b. Being coincidentally shared by two totally different creatures.
c. Being inherited by the organisms' common ancestors.
d. Mutating beyond all reasonable expectations.

5. The manner in which instructions for building proteins, the basic structural molecules of living material are written in the DNA, is

a. Genotypic assignment.
b. Chromosome pattern.
c. Genetic code.
d. Genetic fingerprinting.

6. A _____ is a unit of inherited material, encoded by a strand of DNA and transcribed by RNA.

   a. Allele
   b. Phenotype
   c. Gene
   d. Genotype

7. Which, if any, of the following statements about meiosis are correct?

   a. During meiosis, the number of chromosomes in the cell are halved.
   b. Meiosis only occurs in eukaryotic cells.
   c. Meiosis is the part of the life cycle that involves sexual reproduction.
   d. All of these statements are correct.

8. A population of wolves expanded exponentially after a hunting ban. Within a few generations, their habitat exceeded its _____ _____.

   a. Carrying capacity
   b. Food source
   c. Population limit
   d. Supply capability

9. When a pouch in the large intestine becomes inflamed, this becomes an affliction known as

   a. Diverticulosis.
   b. Diverticulitis.
   c. Acid Reflux.
   d. Colon Cancer.

10. Why is detection of pathogens complicated?

    a. They evolve so quickly
    b. They die so quickly
    c. They are invisible
    d. They multiply so quickly

Practice Test Questions Set 1

11. Photosynthesis is

    a. The process by which plants generate oxygen from carbon dioxide.

    b. The process by which plants generate carbon dioxide from oxygen.

    c. The process by which plants generate carbon dioxide and oxygen.

    d. None of the above.

12. Which, if any, of the following statements are false?

    a. A mutation is a permanent change in the DNA sequence of a gene.

    b. Mutations in a gene's DNA sequence can alter the amino acid sequence of the protein encoded by the gene.

    c. Mutations in DNA sequences usually occur spontaneously.

    d. Mutations in DNA sequences is caused by exposure to environmental agents such as sunshine.

13. Starting with the weakest, arrange the fundamental forces of nature in order of strength.

    a. Gravity, Weak Nuclear Force, Electromagnetic Force, Strong Nuclear Force

    b. Weak Nuclear Force, Gravity, Electromagnetic Force, Strong Nuclear Force

    c. Strong Nuclear Force, Weak Nuclear Force, Electromagnetic Force, Gravity

    d. Gravity, Strong Nuclear Force, Weak Nuclear Force, Electromagnetic Force

14. _____, which refers to the repeatability of measurement, does not require knowledge of the correct or true value.

    a. Precision

    b. Value

    c. Certainty

    d. Accuracy

15. Artificial selection

    a. Is a process where desirable traits are systematically bred.

    b. Is a process where traits become more or less common in a population.

    c. Is a process where behaviors are favored.

    d. None of the above.

16. Which of the following are not examples of vaporization?

a. Boiling
b. Evaporation
c. Condensation
d. All of the above

17. Describe the periodic table.

a. The periodic table is a tabular display of the chemical compounds organized on the basis of their atomic numbers, electron configurations, and recurring chemical properties.
b. The periodic table is a tabular display of the chemical elements, organized on the basis of their atomic numbers, electron configurations, and recurring chemical properties.
c. The periodic table is a tabular display of the chemical subatomic particles, organized on the basis of their atomic numbers, electron configurations, and recurring chemical properties.
d. None of the above.

18. In terms of the scientific method, the term _____ refers to the act of noticing or perceiving something and/or recording a fact or occurrence.

a. Observation
b. Diligence
c. Perception
d. Control

19. What is the difference, of any, between kinetic energy and potential energy?

a. Kinetic energy is the energy of a body resulting from heat while potential energy is the energy possessed by an object that is chilled.
b. Kinetic energy is the energy of a body resulting from motion while potential energy is the energy possessed by an object by virtue of its position or state, e.g., as in a compressed spring.
c. There is no difference between kinetic and potential energy; all energy is the same.
d. Potential energy is the energy of a body resulting from motion while kinetic energy is the energy possessed by an object by virtue of its position or state, e.g., as in a compressed spring.

Practice Test Questions Set 1

20. What is the sequence of developmental stages through which members of a given species must pass?

    a. Life cycle

    b. Life expectancy

    c. Life sequence

    d. None of the above

21. Which one of the following best describes the function of a cell membrane?

    a. It controls the substances entering and leaving the cell.

    b. It keeps the cell in shape.

    c. It controls the substances entering the cell.

    d. It supports the cell structures.

22. Which of these is not a rank within the area of classification or taxonomy?

    a. Species

    b. Family

    c. Genus

    d. Relative position

23. A _____ is a statistic used as a measure of the dispersion or variation in a distribution.

    a. Normal distribution

    b. Range

    c. Outlier

    d. Standard deviation

24. Substances that deactivate catalysts are called

    a. Inhibitors.

    b. Catalytic poisons.

    c. Positive catalysts.

    d. None of the above.

25. Describe kinetic energy.

a. Kinetic energy is the energy an object possesses due to its mass.

b. Kinetic energy is the energy an object possesses due to its motion.

c. Kinetic energy is the energy an object possesses due to its chemical properties.

d. Kinetic energy is the stored energy an object possesses.

26. The interval of confidence around the measured value, such that the measured value is certain not to lie outside this stated interval, refers to the _____ of that value.

a. Accuracy

b. Error

c. Uncertainty

d. Measurement

27. What are the differences, if any, between arteries, veins, and capillaries?

a. Veins carry oxygenated blood away from the heart, arteries return oxygen-depleted blood to the heart, and capillaries are thin-walled blood vessels in which gas/ nutrient/ waste exchange occurs.

b. Capillaries carry oxygenated blood away from the heart, veins return oxygen-depleted blood to the heart, and capillaries are thin-walled blood vessels in which gas/ nutrient/ waste exchange occurs.

c. There are no differences; all perform the same function in different parts of the body.

d. Arteries carry oxygenated blood away from the heart, veins return oxygen-depleted blood to the heart, and capillaries are thin-walled blood vessels in which gas/ nutrient/ waste exchange occurs.

28. What part of the body starts inhalation?

a. The lungs

b. The diaphragm

c. The larynx

d. The kidneys

29. Another term for biological classification is:

a. Darwinian classification.

b. Animal classification.

c. Molecular classification.

d. Scientific classification.

Practice Test Questions Set 1

30. What type of gene is not expressed as a trait unless inherited by both parents?

    a. Principal gene

    b. Latent gene

    c. Recessive gene

    d. Dominant gene

31. A _____ _____ is an approximation or simulation of a real system that omits all but the most essential variables of the system.

    a. Scientific method

    b. Independent variable

    c. Control group

    d. Scientific model

32. Neutrons are necessary within an atomic nucleus because

    a. They bind with protons via nuclear force.

    b. They bind with nuclei via nuclear force.

    c. They bind with protons via electromagnetic force.

    d. They bind with nuclei via electromagnetic force.

33. Which of the following statements is false?

    a. Most enzymes are proteins

    b. Enzymes are catalysts

    c. Most enzymes are inorganic

    d. Enzymes are large biological molecules

34. _____ are compounds that contain hydrogen, can dissolve in water to release hydrogen ions into solution, and, in an aqueous solution, can conduct electricity.

    a. Caustics

    b. Bases

    c. Acids

    d. Salts

35. What are the basic structural units of nucleic acids (DNA or RNA) whose sequence determines individual hereditary characteristics?

   a. Gene
   b. Nucleotide
   c. Phosphate
   d. Nitrogen base

36. List the classifications of organisms in order of size.

   a. Genus, Kingdom, Phylum/division, Class, Order, and Family Species
   b. Order, Kingdom, Phylum/division, Genus, Class, and Family Species
   c. Genus, Kingdom, Phylum/division, Class, Order, and Family Species
   d. Kingdom ,Genus, Phylum/division, Class, Order, and Family Species
   e. Family species, Order, Class, Phylum/division, Kingdom, and Genus

37. Where does digestion begin?

   a. In the throat
   b. In the stomach
   c. In the intestines
   d. In the mouth

38. What are the main components of the circulatory system?

   a. The heart, veins and blood vessels
   b. The heart, brain, and ears
   c. The nose, throat and ears
   d. The lungs, stomach, and kidneys

39. What is an example of a pathogen that the immune system detects?

   a. An atom
   b. A molecule
   c. A vitamin
   d. A virus

Practice Test Questions Set 1

40. Explain chemical bonds.

a. Chemical bonds are attractions between atoms that form chemical substances containing two or more atoms.

b. Chemical bonds are attractions between protons that form chemical elements containing two or more atoms.

c. Chemical bonds are two or more atoms that form chemical substances.

d. None of the above.

41. Which of these is not an example of a function of the stomach in digestion?

a. Storing food

b. Cleansing food of impurities

c. Mixing food with digestive juices

d. Transferring food into the intestines

42. The exchange of oxygen for carbon dioxide takes place in the alveolar area of

a. The throat.

b. The ears.

c. The appendix.

d. The lungs.

43. The number of protons in the nucleus of an atom is the

a. Atomic mass.

b. Atomic weight.

c. Atomic number.

d. None of the above.

44. Natural selection is

a. A process where biological traits become more common in a population.

b. A process where biological traits become less common in a population.

c. A process where biological traits become more or less common in a population.

d. None of the above.

45. Sex chromosomes are designated as being "X" or "Y" chromosomes. In terms of sex chromosomes, what differences exist between males and females?

   a. Females have two X chromosomes and males have one X chromosome and one Y chromosome.

   b. Females have one X chromosome, and males have one X chromosome and one Y chromosome.

   c. Females have one Y chromosome, while males have one X chromosome.

   d. Females have one X chromosome and one Y chromosome, and males have two X chromosomes.

46. How does the immune system fight off disease?

   a. By identifying and killing tumor cells and pathogens.

   b. By creating new blood cells that fight disease.

   c. By expelling infection through the blood stream.

   d. By giving you energy to resist disease infections.

47. Identify the chemical properties of water.

   a. Water has two hydrogen atoms covalently bonded to one oxygen atom.

   b. Water has two oxygen atoms covalently bonded to one hydrogen atom.

   c. Water has two hydrogen atoms polar covalently bonded to one oxygen atom.

   d. Water has two oxygen atoms polar covalently bonded to one hydrogen atom.

48. Which of the following is not true of atomic theory?

   a. Originated in the early 19th century with the work of John Dalton.

   b. Is the field of physics that describes the characteristics and properties of atoms that make up matter.

   c. Explains temperature as the momentum of atoms.

   d. Explains macroscopic phenomena through the behavior of microscopic atoms.

Practice Test 1 - Quick Reference Answer Key

Section 1 – Reading

1. A
2. B
3. A
4. B
5. D
6. B
7. C
8. A
9. B
10. A
11. A
12. A
13. C
14. B
15. A
16. C
17. C
18. C
19. D
20. C
21. C
22. C
23. B
24. D
25. B
26. B
27. C
28. A
29. D
30. B
31. C
32. A
33. C
34. D
35. A

Section II – Math

1. A
2. D
3. D
4. B
5. C
6. C
7. A
8. A
9. B
10. A
11. B
12. D
13. B
14. A
15. C
16. B
17. A
18. B
19. C
20. C
21. D
22. C
23. D
24. D
25. B
26. B
27. B
28. B
29. A
30. D

Section III English

1. A
2. A
3. B
4. C
5. A
6. A
7. C
8. D
9. B
10. A
11. A
12. D

13. B
14. D
15. C
16. A
17. A
18. A
19. A
20. A
21. B
22. C
23. B
24. B
25. A
26. B
27. B
28. B
29. D
30. B

28. B
29. D
30. C
31. D
32. A
33. C
34. C
35. A
36. A
37. D
38. A
39. D
40. A
41. B
42. D
43. C
44. C
45. A
46. A
47. A
48. C

Section IV – Science

1. A
2. A
3. A
4. C
5. C
6. C
7. D
8. A
9. B
10. A
11. A
12. C
13. A
14. A
15. A
16. C
17. B
18. A
19. B
20. A
21. A
22. D
23. D
24. B
25. B
26. C
27. D

Answer Key with Explanations

Section 1 – Reading

1. A
Helen's parents hired Anne to teach Helen to communicate. Choice B is incorrect because the passage states Anne had trouble finding her way around, which means she could walk. Choice C is incorrect because you don't hire a teacher to teach someone to play. Choice D is incorrect because by age 6, if Helen had never eaten, she would have starved to death.

2. B
The correct answer because that fact is stated directly in the passage. The passage explains that Anne taught Helen to hear by allowing her to feel the vibrations in her throat.

3. A
We can infer that Anne is a patient teacher because she did not leave or lose her temper when Helen bit or hit her; she just kept trying to teach Helen. Choice B is incorrect because Anne taught Helen to read and talk. Choice C is incorrect because Anne could hear. She was partially blind, not deaf. Choice D is incorrect because it does not have to do with patience.

4. B
The passage states that it was hard for anyone but Anne to understand Helen when she spoke. Choice A is incorrect because the passage does not mention Helen spoke a foreign language. Choice C is incorrect because there is no mention of how quiet or loud Helen's voice was. Choice D is incorrect because we know from reading the passage that Helen did learn to speak.

5. D
This question tests the reader's summarization skills. The question is asking very generally about the message of the passage, and the title, "Ways Characters Communicate in Theater," is one indication of that. The other choices A, B, and C are all directly from the text, and therefore readers may be inclined to select one of them, but are too specific to encapsulate the entirety of the passage and its message.

6. B
The paragraph on soliloquies mentions "To be or not to be," and it is from the context of that paragraph that readers may understand that because "To be or not to be" is a soliloquy, Hamlet will be introspective, or thoughtful, while delivering it. It is true that actors deliver soliloquies alone, and may be "solitary" (choice A), but "thoughtful" (choice B) is more true to the overall idea of the paragraph. Readers may choose C because drama and theater can be used interchangeably and the passage mentions that soliloquies are

unique to theater (and therefore drama), but this answer is not specific enough to the paragraph in question. Readers may pick up on the theme of life and death and Hamlet's true intentions and select that he is "hopeless" (choice D), but those themes are not discussed either by this paragraph or passage, as a close textual reading and analysis confirms.

7. C
This question tests the reader's grammatical skills. Choice B seems logical, but parenthesis are actually considered to be a stronger break in a sentence than commas are, and along this line of thinking, actually disrupt the sentence more.

Choices A and D make comparisons between theater and film that are simply not made in the passage, and may or may not be true. This detail does clarify the statement that asides are most unique to theater by adding that it is not completely unique to theater, which may have been why the author didn't chose not to delete it and instead used parentheses to designate the detail's importance (choice C).

8. A
Low blood sugar occurs both in diabetics and healthy adults.

9. B
None of the statements are the author's opinion.

10. A
The author's purpose is the inform.

11. A
The only statement that is not a detail is, "A doctor can diagnosis this medical condition by asking the patient questions and testing."

12. A
This sentence is a recommendation.

13. C
Tips for a good night's sleep is the best alternative title for this article.

14. B
Mental activity is helpful for a good night's sleep is can not be inferred from this article.

15. A
From the passage, one disadvantage of taking naps is they may keep you awake at night.

16. C
Based on the partial table of contents, you would find information about natural selection in the ecology section on page 110.

17. C
To be infamous means to be remembered for an evil or terrible action. Therefore, the word infamy means to remember a bad or terrible thing. Choice A is incorrect because

being famous is not the same as being infamous. Choice B is incorrect because the attack on Pearl Harbor was not good. Choice D is incorrect because Pearl Harbor was not forgotten.

18. C
Each other answer set contains the name of at least one country that was not part of the AXIS powers.

19. D
It is stated in the passage. Choice A is not correct because there was no indication that Japan would attack San Diego
Choice B is incorrect because the attack on Pearl Harbor was a surprise. Choice C is incorrect because Roosevelt was not planning to attack Japan.

20. C
The passage clearly states that Japan planned a surprise attack. They chose that early time to catch the U.S. military off guard. Choice A is incorrect because the military does not sleep late. Choice B is incorrect because there is no law against bombing countries. Choice D is incorrect because it makes no sense.

21. C
This question tests the reader's vocabulary skills. The uses of the negatives "but" and "less," especially right next to each other, may confuse readers into answering with choices A or D, which list words that are antonyms to "militant." Readers may also be confused by the comparison of healthy people with what is being described as an overly healthy person--both people are good, but the reader may look for which one is "worse" in the comparison, and therefore stray toward the antonym words. One key to understanding the meaning of "militant" if the reader is unfamiliar with it is to look at the root of the word; readers can then easily associate it with "military" and gain a sense of what the word signifies: defence (especially considered that the immune system defends the body). Choice C is correct over choice B because "militant" is an adjective, just as the words in choice C are, whereas the words in choice B are nouns.

22. C
This question tests the reader's understanding of function within writing. The other choices are details included surrounding the quoted text, and may therefore confuse the reader. Choice A somewhat contradicts what is said earlier in the paragraph, which is that tests and treatments are improving, and probably doctors are along with them, but the paragraph doesn't actually mention doctors, and the subject of the question is the medicine. Choice B may seem correct to readers who aren't careful to understand that, while the author does mention the large number of people affected, the author is touching on the realities of living with allergies rather about the likelihood of curing all allergies. Similarly, while the author does mention the "balance" of the body, which is easily associated with "wholesome," the author is not really making an argument and especially is not making an extreme statement that allergy medicines should be outlawed. Again, because the article's tone is on living with allergies, choice C is an appropriate choice that fits with the title and content of the text.

23. B

This question tests the reader's inference skills. The text does not state who is doing the recommending, but the use of the "patients," as well as the general context of the passage, lends itself to the logical partner, "doctors," choice B. The author does mention the recommendation but doesn't present it as her own (i.e. "I recommend that"), so choice A may be eliminated. It may seem plausible that people with allergies (choice D) may recommend medicines or products to other people with allergies, but the text does not necessarily support this interaction taking place. Choice C may be selected because the EpiPen is specifically mentioned, but the use of the phrase "such as" when it is introduced is not limiting enough to assume the recommendation is coming from its creators.

24. D

This question tests the reader's global understanding of the text. Choice D includes the main topics of the three body paragraphs, and isn't too focused on a specific aspect or quote from the text, as the other questions are, giving a skewed summary of what the author intended. The reader may be drawn to choice B because of the title of the passage and the use of words like "better," but the message of the passage is larger and more general than this.

25. B

Reading the document posted to the Human Resources website is optional.

26. B

The document is recommended changes and have not be implemented yet.

27. C

This question tests the reader's summarization skills. The use of the word "actually" in describing what kind of people poets are, as well as other moments like this, may lead readers to selecting choices B or D, but the author is more information than trying to persuade readers. The author gives no indication that she loves poetry (choice B) or that people, students specifically (D), should write poems. Choice A is incorrect because the style and content of this paragraph do not match those of a foreword; forewords usually focus on the history or ideas of a specific poem to introduce it more fully and help it stand out against other poems. The author here focuses on several poems and gives broad statements. Instead, she tells a kind of story about poems, giving three very broad time periods in which to discuss them, thereby giving a brief history of poetry, as choice C states.

28. A

This question tests the reader's summarization skills. Key words in the topic sentences of each of the paragraphs ("oldest," "Renaissance," "modern") should give the reader an idea that the author is moving chronologically. The opening and closing sentence-paragraphs are broad and talk generally. B seems reasonable, but epic poems are mentioned in two paragraphs, eliminating the idea that only new types of poems are used in each paragraph. Choice C is also easily eliminated because the author clearly mentions several different poets, groups of people, and poems. Choice D also seems reasonable, considering that the author does move from older forms of poetry to newer forms, but use of "so (that)" makes this statement false, for the author gives no indication that she is rushing (the paragraphs are about the same size) or that she prefers modern poetry.

29. D
This question tests the reader's attention to detail. The key word is "invented"-- it ties together the Mesopotamians, who invented the written word, and the fact that they, as the inventors, also invented and used poetry. The other selections focus on other details mentioned in the passage, such as that the Renaissance's admiration of the Greeks (choice C) and that Beowulf is in Old English (choice A). Choice B may seem like an attractive answer because it is unlike the others and because the idea of heroes seems rooted in ancient and early civilizations.

30. B
This question tests the reader's vocabulary and contextualization skills. "Telling" is not an unusual word, but it may be used here in a way that is not familiar to readers, as an adjective rather than a verb in gerund form. A may seem like the obvious answer to a reader looking for a verb to match the use they are familiar with. If the reader understands that the word is being used as an adjective and that choice A is a ploy, they may opt to select choice D, "wordy," but it does not make sense in context. Choice C can be easily eliminated, and doesn't have any connection to the paragraph or passage. "Significant" (choice B) makes sense contextually, especially relative to the phrase "give insight" used later in the sentence.

31. C
Wind is the highest source of renewable energy in Scotland. The other choices are either not mentioned at all or not mentioned in the context for how fast they are growing.

32. A
Most Scottish citizens agree with the Government's plan due to the concern for current and future needs.

Choice B is a good choice but not why the majority agree. Choice C is meant to mislead the as they are clearly in sight. Choice D is a good 'common sense' choice but mentioned specifically in the text.

33. C
The up-front cost is expensive.
The other choices may appear to be correct, and even be common sense, but they are not specifically mentioned in the paragraph.

34. D
The best way to describe the paragraphs description of wind energy is clean and renewable but fluctuating.
The other choices are good descriptions of wind energy, but not the best way to describe the article.

35. A
The Save the Children's fund has raised $12,000 out of $20,000, or 12/20. Simplifying, 12/20 = 3/5

Section II – Math

1. A
1/3 X 3/4 = 3/12 = 1/4
To multiply fractions, multiply the numerator and denominator.

2. D
The question asks for approximate cost, so work with round numbers. The jacket costs $545.00 so we can round up to $550. 10% of $550 is 55. We can round down to $50, which is easier to work with. $550 - $50 is $500. The jacket will cost about $500.

The actual cost will be 10% X 545 = $54.50
545 – 54.50 = $490.50

3. D
3.14 + 2.73 = 5.87 and 5.87 + 23.7 = 29.57

4. B
Spent 15%, so 100% - 15% = 85%

5. C
To convert a decimal to a fraction, take the places of decimal as your denominator, here, 2, so in 0.27, '7' is in the 100th place, so the fraction is 27/100 and 0.33 becomes 33/100.

Next estimate the answer quickly to eliminate obvious wrong choices. 27/100 is about 1/4 and 33/100 is 1/3. 1/3 is slightly larger than 1/4, and 1/4 + 1/4 is 1/2, so the answer will be slightly larger than 1/2.
Looking at the choices, Choice A can be eliminated since 3/6 = 1/2. Choice D, 2/7 is less than 1/2 and be eliminated. The answer is going to be Choice B or Choice C.

Do the calculation, 0.27 + 0.33 = 0.60 and 0.60 = 60/100 = 3/5, Choice C is correct.

6. C
This is an easy question, and shows how you can solve some questions without doing the calculations. The question is, 8 is what percent of 40. Take easy percentages for an approximate answer and see what you get.

10% is easy to calculate because you can drop the zero, or move the decimal point.
10% of 40 = 4, and 8 = 2 X 4, so, 8 must be 2 X 10% = 20%.

Here are the calculations which confirm the quick approximation.
8/40 = X/100 = 8 * 100 / 40X = 800/40 = X = 20

7. A
According to the graph, oil consumption peaked in 2011.

Practice Test Questions Set 1

8. A
2 + a number divided by 7.
(2 + X) divided by 7.
(2 + X)/7

9. B
.4/100 * 36 = .4 * 36/100 = .144

10. A
5 mg/10/mg X 1 tab/1 = .5 tablets

11. B
Step 1: Set up the formula to calculate the dose to be given in mg as per weight of the child:- Dose ordered X Weight in Kg = Dose to be given
Step 2: 20 mg X 12 kg = 240 mg
240 mg/80 mg X 1 tab/1 = 240/80 = 3 tablets

12. D
Indonesia is growing the fastest at about 30%.

13. B
$(4)(3)^3 = (4)(27) = 108$

14. A
MCMXC is 1990. 1000 + (1000 − 100) + (100 − 10) = 1990

15. C
4 quarts = 1 gallon, 16 quarts = 16/4 = 4 gallons. Conversion problems are easy to get confused. One way to think of them is which is larger - quarts or gallons? Gallons are larger, so if you are converting from quarts to gallons the number of gallons will be a smaller number. Keeping that in mind, you can do a 'common-sense' check your answer.

16. B
0.45 kg = 1 pound, 1 kg. = 1/0.45 and 45 kg = 1/0.45 x 45 = 99.208, or 100 pounds.

17. A
Three plus a number times 7 equals 42. Let X be the number.
(3 + X) times 7 = 42
7(3 + X) = 42

18. B
Number of absent students = 83 − 72 = 11

Percentage of absent students is found by proportioning the number of absent students to total number of students in the class = 11•100/83 = 13.25

Checking the answers, we round 13.25 to the nearest whole number: 13%

19. C
To solve for x, first simplify the equation
5x + 2x + 14 = 14x – 7
7x - 14x = -14 -7
-7x = -21
x = -21/-7
x = 3

20. C
5z + 5 = 3z + 6 + 11
5z -3z + 5 = 6 + 11
5z – 3z = 6 + 11 -5
2z = 17 – 5
2z = 12
z = 12/2
z = 6

21. D
Price increased by $5 ($25-$20). To calculate the percent increase:
5/20 = X/100
500 = 20X
X = 500/20
X = 25%

22. C
The ratio is 2 to 8, or 1:4.

23. D
2 glasses are broken for 43 customers so 1 glass breaks for every 43/2 customers served, therefore 10 glasses implies (43/2)•10 = 215 customers.

24. D
As the lawn is square , the length of one side will be the square root of the area. √62,500 = 250 meters. So, the perimeter is found by 4 times the length of the side of the square:

250•4 = 1000 meters.

Since each meter costs $5.5, the total cost of the fence will be 1000•5.5 = $5,500.

25. B
5n + (19 – 2) = 67, 5n + 17 = 67, 5n = 67 -17, 5n = 50, n = 50/5 = 10

26. B

Day	Absent	Present	%
Monday	5	40	88.88%
Tuesday	9	36	80.00%
Wednesday	4	41	91.11%

| Thursday | 10 | 35 | 77.77% |
| Friday | 6 | 39 | 86.66% |

Sum of the percent attendance is 424.42. Divide by 5 for the average, 424.42/5 = 84.884. Round up to 85%.

27. B

The distribution is done in three different rates and amounts:

$6.4 per 20 kilograms to 15 shops ... 20•15 = 300 kilograms distributed

$3.4 per 10 kilograms to 12 shops ... 10•12 = 120 kilograms distributed

550 - (300 + 120) = 550 - 420 = 130 kilograms left. This amount is distributed by 5 kilogram portions. So, this means that there are 130/5 = 26 shops.

$1.8 per 130 kilograms.

We need to find the amount he earned overall these distributions.

$6.4 per 20 kilograms : 6.4•15 = $96 for 300 kilograms

$3.4 per 10 kilograms : 3.4•12 = $40.8 for 120 kilograms

$1.8 per 5 kilograms : 1.8•26 = $46.8 for 130 kilograms

So, he earned 96 + 40.8 + 46.8 = $ 183.6

The total distribution cost is given as $10

The profit is found by: Money earned - money spent ... It is important to remember that he bought 550 kilograms of potatoes for $165 at the beginning:

Profit = 183.6 - 10 - 165 = $8.6

28. B

We check the fractions taking place in the question. We see that there is a "half" (that is 1/2) and 3/7. So, we multiply the denominators of these fractions to decide how to name the total money. We say that Mr. Johnson has 14x at the beginning; he gives half of this, meaning 7x, to his family. $250 to his landlord. He has 3/7 of his money left. 3/7 of 14x is equal to:

14x•(3/7) = 6x

So,

Spent money is: 7x + 250

Unspent money is: 6x

Total money is: 14x

We write an equation: total money = spent money + unspent money

14x = 7x + 250 + 6x

14x - 7x - 6x = 250

x = 250

We are asked to find the total money that is 14x:

14x = 14•250 = $3500

29. A
The probability that the 1st ball drawn is red = 4/11
The probability that the 2nd ball drawn is green = 5/10
The combined probability will then be 4/11 X 5/10 = 20/110 = 2/11

30. D
First calculate total square feet, which is 15 * 24 = 360 ft^2. Next, convert this value to square yards, (1 yards^2 = 9 ft^2) which is 360/9 = 40 yards^2. At $0.50 per square yard, the total cost is 40 * 0.50 = $20.

Section III English

1. A
The third conditional is used for talking about an unreal situation (a situation that did not happen) in the past. For example, "If I had studied harder, [if clause] I would have passed the exam" [main clause]. This has the same meaning as, "I failed the exam, because I didn't study hard enough."

2. A
Use a plural verb form for two subjects linked by "and."

3. B
In double negative sentences, one negative is replaced with "any."

4. C
"It's" is a contraction for it is or it has. "Its" is a possessive pronoun.

5. A
When two subjects are linked by "with" or "as well," use the verb form that matches the first subject.

6. A
The sentence requires the past perfect "has always been known." This is the only grammatically correct choice.

7. C

Practice Test Questions Set 1

The superlative, "hottest," is used when expressing a temperature greater than that of anything to which it is being compared.

8. D
When comparing two items, use "the taller." When comparing more than two items, use "the tallest."

9. B
The past perfect form is used to describe an event that occurred in the past and prior to another event. Here there are two things that happened, both of them in the past, and something the person wanted to do.

Event 1: Kiss came to town
Event 2: All the tickets sold out
What I wanted to do: Buy a ticket

The events are arranged:
When KISS came to town, all the tickets **had been sold out** before I could buy one.

10. A
The subject is "rules" so the present tense plural form, "are," is used to agree with "realize."

11. A
"Who" is correct because the question uses an active construction. "To whom was first place given?" is a passive construction.

12. D
"Which" is correct, because the files are objects and not people.

13. B
Use a singular verb with either, each, neither, everyone and many.

14. D
Maintenance is the correct spelling.

15. C
Humorous is the correct spelling.

16. A
Mathematics is the correct spelling.

17. A
Use a comma to separate phrases.

18. A
The Sahara Desert is a proper name so capitalized. The names of countries, ie Africa are capitalized.

19. A
'She' is the simple subject of this sentence.

20. A
The simple predicate is 'studied long and hard.' The predicate of a sentence is the action performed by the subject.

21. B
This is an interrogative sentence.

22. C
It is not necessary to say the fish came from the topics, since we already know they are tropical.

23. B
The correct sentence is
Historians have been guessing for more than 100 years the doctor was a woman.

Here the phrase 'for more than 100 years' refers to how long historians have been guessing, and not to how long the doctor has been a woman.

24. B
Use a comma separates independent clauses. None of us wants to go to the party, not even if there will be live music.

25. A
This is an example where a comma appears before 'and,' but is disambiguating. Without the comma, the sentence would be "I own two dogs, a cat named Jeffrey and Henry, the goldfish." This means there is a cat named Jeffrey and Henry, and a goldfish with no name mentioned. The comma appears to show the distinction.

I own two dogs, a cat named Jeffrey, and Henry, the goldfish.

26. B
President is not capitalized unless used with a name as in, President Obama.

27. B
'Jumped' is a verb. Verbs describe an action, state, or occurrence.

28. B
A confrontation is a head-on conflict, so a direct confrontation is redundant.

29. D
Pesticide: NOUN a substance, usually synthetic although sometimes biological, used to kill or contain the activities of pests.

30. B
Hormones: NOUN any substance produced by one tissue and conveyed by the bloodstream to another to effect physiological activity.

Practice Test Questions Set 1

Section IV – Science

1. A
Phenotype refers to observed properties of an organism and genotype refers to the genes of an organism.

2. A
A solution with a pH value of greater than 7 is base.

3. A
Eukaryotic and prokaryotic cells are both organelles.

4. C
Homologous is being inherited by the organisms' common ancestors. An example would be feathers and hair—both of which were structures that shared a common ancestral trait.

5. C
The manner in which instructions for building proteins, the basic structural molecules of living material are written in the DNA is a **genetic code**.

6. C
A gene is a unit of inherited material, encoded by a strand of DNA and transcribed by RNA.

7. D
All these statements are correct.

  a. During meiosis, the number of chromosomes in the cell are halved.
  b. Meiosis only occurs in eukaryotic cells.
  c. Meiosis is the part of the life cycle that involves sexual reproduction.

8. A Carrying capacity
An area's carrying capacity is the maximum number of animals of a given species that area can support during the harshest part of the year.

9. B
Diverticulitis is a pouch in the large intestine becomes inflamed.

10. A
Detection of pathogens can be complicated because they evolve so quickly.

11. A
Photosynthesis is the process by which plants and other photoautotrophs generate carbohydrates and oxygen from carbon dioxide, water, and light energy in chloroplasts.

12. C

Mutations in DNA sequences usually occur spontaneously is false.

13. A

Starting with the weakest, the fundamental forces of nature in order of strength are, Gravity, Weak nuclear force, Electromagnetic force, Strong nuclear force.

14. A

Precision, which refers to the repeatability of measurement, does not require knowledge of the correct or true value.

15. A

Artificial selection is a process where desirable traits are systematically bred.

16. C

Condensation is not an example of vaporization. Boiling and evaporation are both examples of vaporization. Condensation is the process by which matter transitions from a gas into a liquid.

17. B

The periodic table is a tabular display of the chemical elements, organized by their atomic numbers, electron configurations, and recurring chemical properties.

18. A

In terms of the scientific method, the term observation refers to the act of noticing or perceiving something and/or recording a fact or occurrence.

19. B

Kinetic energy is the energy of a body that results from motion while potential energy is the energy possessed by an object by virtue of its position or state, e.g., as in a compressed spring.

20. A

A life cycle is the sequence of developmental stages through which members of a given species must pass.

21. A

The cell membrane is a biological membrane that separates the interior of all cells from the outside environment. The cell membrane is selectively permeable to ions and organic molecules and controls the movement of substances in and out of cells. [16]

22. D

Relative position. Ranks include Domain, Kingdom, Phylum, Class, Order, Family, Genus, and Species.

23. D

A Standard deviation is a statistic used as a measure of the dispersion or variation in a distribution.

24. B
Substances that deactivate catalysts are called catalytic poisons.

25. B
Kinetic energy is the energy an object possesses due to its motion.

26. C
The interval of confidence around the measured value, such that the measured value is certain not to lie outside the stated interval refers to the **uncertainty** of that value.

27. D
Arteries carry oxygenated blood away from the heart, veins return oxygen-depleted blood to the heart, and capillaries are thin-walled blood vessels in which gas/ nutrient/ waste exchange occurs.

Note: An easy way to remember the difference between an artery and a vein is that Arteries carry Away from the heart.

28. B
The thoracic diaphragm, is a skeletal muscle across the bottom of the rib cage. The thoracic membrane is important in respiratory function.

29. D
Scientific classification. The two phrases are interchangeable, although the former seems to more accurately reflect the purpose of classification: to categorize biological units.

30. C
A recessive gene is not expressed as a trait unless inherited by both parents.

31. D
A scientific model is an approximation or simulation of a real system that omits all but the most essential variables of the system.

32. A
Neutrons are necessary within an atomic nucleus as they bind with protons via the nuclear force.

33. C
The following statement is false - Most enzymes are inorganic.

34. C
Acids are compounds that contain hydrogen and can dissolve in water to release hydrogen ions into solution.

35. A
Genes determine individual hereditary characteristics.

36. A

The groups into which organisms are classified are called taxa and include, in order of size, Genus, Kingdom, Phylum/division, Class, Order, and Family Species.

37. D

Digestion begins in the mouth.

38. A

The main components of the circulatory system are the heart, veins and blood vessels.

39. D

An example of a pathogen that the immune system detects is a virus.

40. A

Chemical bonds are attractions between atoms that form chemical substances containing two or more atoms.

41. B

Cleansing food of impurities is not an example of a function of the stomach in digestion.

42. D

The exchange of oxygen for carbon dioxide takes place in the alveolar area of the lungs.

43. C

In chemistry, the number of protons in the nucleus of an atom is known as the atomic number, which determines the chemical element to which the atom belongs.

44. C

Natural selection is a process where biological traits become more or less common in a population.

45. A

Females have two X chromosomes and males have one X chromosome and one Y chromosome.

46. A

The immune system fight off disease by identifying and killing tumor cells and pathogens.

47. A

Water has two hydrogen atoms covalently bonded to one oxygen atom.

48. C

Choice C (Atomic theory explains temperature as the momentum of atoms.) is incorrect because atomic theory explains temperature as the motion of atoms (faster = hotter), not the momentum. The momentum of atoms explains the outward pressure that they exert.

Practice Test Questions Set 2

Section I – Reading

Questions: 35
Time: 30 Minutes

Section II – Math

Questions: 30
Time: 30 Minutes

Section III – English and Language Usage

Questions: 30
Time: 30 Minutes

Section IV – Science

Questions: 48
Time: 40 Minutes

The questions below are not the same as you will find on the TEAS® - that would be too easy! And nobody knows what the questions will be and they change all the time. Below are general questions that cover the same subject areas as the TEAS®. While the format and exact wording of the questions may differ slightly, and change from year to year, if you can answer the questions below, you will have no problem with the TEAS®.

For the best results, take these practice test questions as if it were the real exam. Set aside times when you will not be disturbed, and a location that is quiet and free of distractions. Read the instructions carefully, read each question carefully, and answer to the best of your ability.

You are given 209 minutes to complete the full TEAS® exam.

Use the bubble answer sheets provided. When you have completed the practice test questions, check your answer against the Answer Key and read the explanation provided.

Do not attempt more than one set of practice test questions in one day. After completing the first practice test, wait two or three days before attempting the second set of questions.

Section I – Reading Answer Sheet

	A	B	C	D	E		A	B	C	D	E
1	○	○	○	○	○	21	○	○	○	○	○
2	○	○	○	○	○	22	○	○	○	○	○
3	○	○	○	○	○	23	○	○	○	○	○
4	○	○	○	○	○	24	○	○	○	○	○
5	○	○	○	○	○	25	○	○	○	○	○
6	○	○	○	○	○	26	○	○	○	○	○
7	○	○	○	○	○	27	○	○	○	○	○
8	○	○	○	○	○	28	○	○	○	○	○
9	○	○	○	○	○	29	○	○	○	○	○
10	○	○	○	○	○	30	○	○	○	○	○
11	○	○	○	○	○	31	○	○	○	○	○
12	○	○	○	○	○	32	○	○	○	○	○
13	○	○	○	○	○	33	○	○	○	○	○
14	○	○	○	○	○	34	○	○	○	○	○
15	○	○	○	○	○	35	○	○	○	○	○
16	○	○	○	○	○						
17	○	○	○	○	○						
18	○	○	○	○	○						
19	○	○	○	○	○						
20	○	○	○	○	○						

Section II – Math – Answer Sheet

	A	B	C	D	E		A	B	C	D	E
1	○	○	○	○	○	21	○	○	○	○	○
2	○	○	○	○	○	22	○	○	○	○	○
3	○	○	○	○	○	23	○	○	○	○	○
4	○	○	○	○	○	24	○	○	○	○	○
5	○	○	○	○	○	25	○	○	○	○	○
6	○	○	○	○	○	26	○	○	○	○	○
7	○	○	○	○	○	27	○	○	○	○	○
8	○	○	○	○	○	28	○	○	○	○	○
9	○	○	○	○	○	29	○	○	○	○	○
10	○	○	○	○	○	30	○	○	○	○	○
11	○	○	○	○	○						
12	○	○	○	○	○						
13	○	○	○	○	○						
14	○	○	○	○	○						
15	○	○	○	○	○						
16	○	○	○	○	○						
17	○	○	○	○	○						
18	○	○	○	○	○						
19	○	○	○	○	○						
20	○	○	○	○	○						

Section III – English and Language Usage Answer Sheet

	A	B	C	D	E		A	B	C	D	E
1	○	○	○	○	○	21	○	○	○	○	○
2	○	○	○	○	○	22	○	○	○	○	○
3	○	○	○	○	○	23	○	○	○	○	○
4	○	○	○	○	○	24	○	○	○	○	○
5	○	○	○	○	○	25	○	○	○	○	○
6	○	○	○	○	○	26	○	○	○	○	○
7	○	○	○	○	○	27	○	○	○	○	○
8	○	○	○	○	○	28	○	○	○	○	○
9	○	○	○	○	○	29	○	○	○	○	○
10	○	○	○	○	○	30	○	○	○	○	○
11	○	○	○	○	○						
12	○	○	○	○	○						
13	○	○	○	○	○						
14	○	○	○	○	○						
15	○	○	○	○	○						
16	○	○	○	○	○						
17	○	○	○	○	○						
18	○	○	○	○	○						
19	○	○	○	○	○						

Section IV – Science Answer Sheet

1. A B C D
2. A B C D
3. A B C D
4. A B C D
5. A B C D
6. A B C D
7. A B C D
8. A B C D
9. A B C D
10. A B C D
11. A B C D
12. A B C D
13. A B C D
14. A B C D
15. A B C D
16. A B C D
17. A B C D
18. A B C D
19. A B C D
20. A B C D
21. A B C D
22. A B C D
23. A B C D
24. A B C D
25. A B C D
26. A B C D
27. A B C D
28. A B C D
29. A B C D
30. A B C D
31. A B C D
32. A B C D
33. A B C D
34. A B C D
35. A B C D
36. A B C D
37. A B C D
38. A B C D
39. A B C D
40. A B C D
41. A B C D
42. A B C D
43. A B C D
44. A B C D
45. A B C D
46. A B C D
47. A B C D
48. A B C D
49. A B C D
50. A B C D

Section I - Reading

Questions 1 - 4 refer to the following passage.

Passage 1 - The Crusades

In 1095 Pope Urban II proclaimed the First Crusade with the intent and stated goal to restore Christian access to holy places in and around Jerusalem. Over the next 200 years there were 6 major crusades and numerous minor crusades in the fight for control of the "Holy Land." Historians are divided on the real purpose of the Crusades, some believing that it was part of a purely defensive war against Islamic conquest; some see them as part of a long-running conflict at the frontiers of Europe; and others see them as confident, aggressive, papal-led expansion attempts by Western Christendom. The impact of the crusades was profound, and judgment of the Crusaders ranges from laudatory to highly critical. However, all agree that the Crusades and wars waged during those crusades were brutal and often bloody. Several hundred thousand Roman Catholic Christians joined the Crusades, they were Christians from all over Europe.

Europe at the time was under the Feudal System, so while the Crusaders made vows to the Church they also were beholden to their Feudal Lords. This led to the Crusaders not only fighting the Saracen, the commonly used word for Muslim at the time, but also each other for power and economic gain in the Holy Land. This infighting between the Crusaders is why many historians hold the view that the Crusades were simply a front for Europe to invade the Holy Land for economic gain in the name of the Church. Another factor contributing to this theory is that while the army of crusaders marched towards Jerusalem they pillaged the land as they went. The church and feudal Lords vowing to return the land to its original beauty, and inhabitants, this rarely happened though as the Lords often kept the land for themselves. A full 800 years after the Crusades, Pope John Paul II expressed his sorrow for the massacre of innocent people and the lasting damage the Medieval church caused in that area of the World.

1. **What is the tone of this article?**

    a. Subjective

    b. Objective

    c. Persuasive

    d. None of the Above

2. **What can all historians agree on concerning the Crusades?**

    a. It achieved great things

    b. It stabilized the Holy Land

    c. It was bloody and brutal

    d. It helped defend Europe from the Byzantine Empire

3. What impact did the feudal system have on the Crusades

　　a. It unified the Crusaders

　　b. It helped gather volunteers

　　c. It had no effect on the Crusades

　　d. It led to infighting, causing more damage than good

4. What does Saracen mean?

　　a. Muslim

　　b. Christian

　　c. Knight

　　d. Holy Land

Questions 5-8 refer to the following passage.

ABC Electric Warranty

ABC Electric Company warrants that its products are free from defects in material and workmanship. Subject to the conditions and limitations set forth below, ABC Electric will, at its option, either repair or replace any part of its products that prove defective due to improper workmanship or materials.

This limited warranty does not cover any damage to the product from improper installation, accident, abuse, misuse, natural disaster, insufficient or excessive electrical supply, abnormal mechanical or environmental conditions, or any unauthorized disassembly, repair, or modification.

This limited warranty also does not apply to any product on which the original identification information has been altered, or removed, has not been handled or packaged correctly, or has been sold as second-hand.

This limited warranty covers only repair, replacement, refund or credit for defective ABC Electric products, as provided above.

5. I tried to repair my ABC Electric blender, but could not, so can I get it repaired under this warranty?

　　a. Yes, the warranty still covers the blender

　　b. No, the warranty does not cover the blender

　　c. Uncertain. ABC Electric may or may not cover repairs under this warranty

6. My ABC Electric fan is not working. Will ABC Electric provide a new one or repair this one?

   a. ABC Electric will repair my fan

   b. ABC Electric will replace my fan

   c. ABC Electric could either replace or repair my fan can request either a replacement or a repair.

7. My stove was damaged in a flood. Does this warranty cover my stove?

   a. Yes, it is covered.

   b. No, it is not covered.

   c. It may or may not be covered.

   d. ABC Electric will decide if it is covered

8. Which of the following is an example of improper workmanship?

   a. Missing parts

   b. Defective parts

   c. Scratches on the front

   d. None of the above

Questions 9 – 12 refer to the following passage.

Passage 2 - Women and Advertising

Only in the last few generations have media messages been so widespread and so readily seen, heard, and read by so many people. Advertising is an important part of both selling and buying anything from soap to cereal to jeans. For whatever reason, more consumers are women than are men. Media message are subtle but powerful, and more attention has been paid lately to how these message affect women.
Of all the products that women buy, makeup, clothes, and other stylistic or cosmetic products are among the most popular. This means that companies focus their advertising on women, promising them that their product will make her feel, look, or smell better than the next company's product will. This competition has resulted in advertising that is more and more ideal and less and less possible for everyday women. However, because women do look to these ideals and the products they represent as how they can potentially become, many women have developed unhealthy attitudes about themselves when they have failed to become those ideals.

In recent years, more companies have tried to change advertisements to be healthier for women. This includes featuring models of more sizes and addressing a huge outcry against unfair tools such as airbrushing and photo editing. There is debate about what the right balance between real and ideal is, because fashion is also considered art and some changes are made to purposefully elevate fashionable products and signify that they are creative, innovative, and the work of individual people. Artists want their freedom protected as much as women do, and advertising agencies are often caught in the middle.

Some claim that the companies who make these changes are not doing enough. Many people worry that there are still not enough models of different sizes and different ethnicities. Some people claim that companies use this healthier type of advertisement not for the good of women, but because they would like to sell products to the women who are looking for these kinds of messages. This is also a hard balance to find: companies do need to make money, and women do need to feel respected.

While the focus of this change has been on women, advertising can also affect men, and this change will hopefully be a lesson on media for all consumers.

9. The second paragraph states that advertising focuses on women

    a. to shape what the ideal should be

    b. because women buy makeup

    c. because women are easily persuaded

    d. because of the types of products that women buy

10. According to the passage, fashion artists and female consumers are at odds because

    a. there is a debate going on and disagreement drives people apart

    b. both of them are trying to protect their freedom to do something

    c. artists want to elevate their products above the reach of women

    d. women are creative, innovative, individual people

11. The author uses the phrase "for whatever reason" in this passage to

    a. keep the focus of the paragraph on media messages and not on the differences between men and women

    b. show that the reason for this is unimportant

    c. argue that it is stupid that more women are consumers than men

    d. show that he or she is tired of talking about why media messages are important

12. This passage suggests that

    a. advertising companies are still working on making their messages better

    b. all advertising companies seek to be more approachable for women

    c. women are only buying from companies that respect them

    d. artists could stop producing fashionable products if they feel bullied

Questions 13 - 16 refer to the following passage.

FDR, the Treaty of Versailles, and the Fourteen Points

At the conclusion of World War I, those who had won the war and those who were forced to admit defeat welcomed the end of the war and expected that a peace treaty would be signed. The American president, Franklin D. Roosevelt, played an important part in proposing what the agreements should be and did so through his Fourteen Points.
World War I had begun in 1914 when an Austrian archduke was assassinated, leading to a domino effect that pulled the world's most powerful countries into war on a large scale. The war catalyzed the creation and use of deadly weapons that had not previously existed, resulting in a great loss of soldiers on both sides of the fighting. More than 9 million soldiers were killed.

The United States agreed to enter the war right before it ended, and many believed that its decision to become finally involved brought on the end of the war. FDR made it very clear that the U.S. was entering the war for moral reasons and had an agenda focused on world peace. The Fourteen Points were individual goals and ideas (focused on peace, free trade, open communication, and self reliance) that FDR wanted the power nations to strive for now that the war had concluded. He was optimistic and had many ideas about what could be accomplished through and during the post-war peace. However, FDR's fourteen points were poorly received when he presented them to the leaders of other world powers, many of whom wanted only to help their own countries and to punish the Germans for fueling the war, and they fell by the wayside. World War II was imminent, for Germany lost everything.

Some historians believe that the other leaders who participated in the Treaty of Versailles weren't receptive to the Fourteen Points because World War I was fought almost entirely on European soil, and the United States lost much less than did the other powers. FDR was in a unique position to determine the fate of the war, but doing it on his own terms did not help accomplish his goals. This is only one historical example of how the United State has tried to use its power as an important country, but found itself limited because of geological or ideological factors.

13. The main idea of this passage is that

    a. World War I was unfair because no fighting took place in America

    b. World War II happened because of the Treaty of Versailles

    c. the power the United States has to help other countries also prevents it from helping other countries

    d. Franklin D. Roosevelt was one of the United States' smartest presidents

14. According to the second paragraph, World War I started because

   a. an archduke was assassinated
   b. weapons that were more deadly had been developed
   c. a domino effect of allies agreeing to help each other
   d. the world's most powerful countries were large

15. The author includes the detail that 9 million soldiers were killed

   a. to demonstrate why European leaders were hesitant to accept peace
   b. to show the reader the dangers of deadly weapons
   c. to make the reader think about which countries lost the most soldiers
   d. to demonstrate why World War II was imminent

16. According to this passage, it can be understood that the word catalyzed means

   a. analyzed
   b. sped up
   c. invented

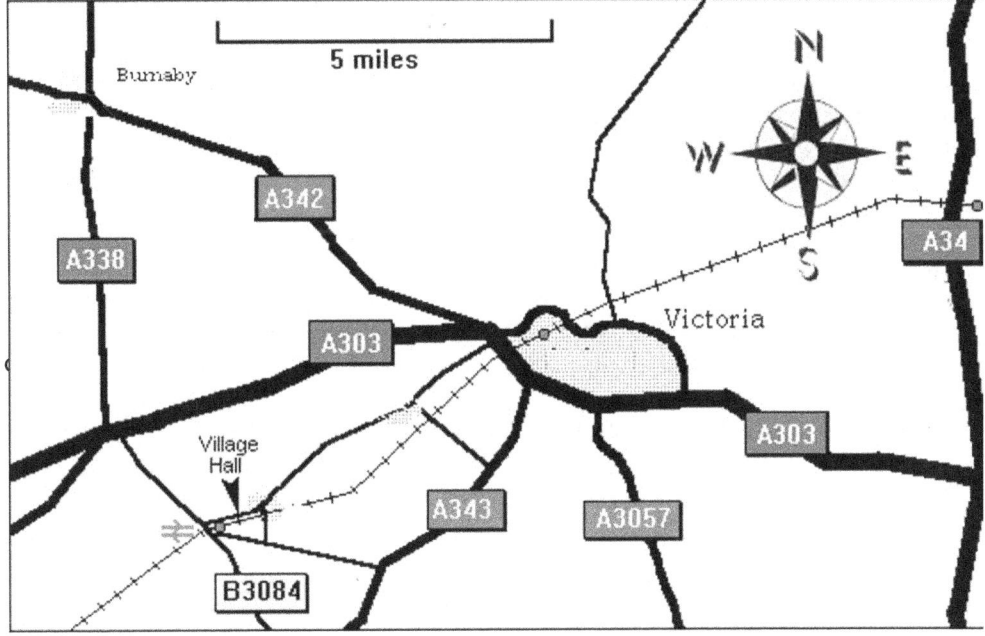

17. **Approximately how far is Victoria to Burnaby?**

    a. About 10 miles
    b. About 5 miles
    c. About 15 miles
    d. About 20 miles

18. **How is the Village Hall from Victoria?**

    a. About 10 miles
    b. About 5 miles
    c. About 15 miles
    d. About 20 miles

Questions 19 - 23 refer to the following passage.

Chocolate Chip Cookies

3/4 cup sugar
3/4 cup packed brown sugar
1 cup butter, softened
2 large eggs, beaten
1 teaspoon vanilla extract
2 1/4 cups all-purpose flour
1 teaspoon baking soda
3/4 teaspoon salt
2 cups semisweet chocolate chips
If desired, 1 cup chopped pecans, or chopped walnuts.
Preheat oven to 375 degrees.

Mix sugar, brown sugar, butter, vanilla and eggs in a large bowl. Stir in flour, baking soda, and salt. The dough will be very stiff.

Stir in chocolate chips by hand with a sturdy wooden spoon. Add the pecans, or other nuts, if desired. Stir until the chocolate chips and nuts are evenly dispersed.

Drop dough by rounded tablespoonfuls 2 inches apart onto a cookie sheet.

Bake 8 to 10 minutes or until light brown. Cookies may look underdone, but they will finish cooking after you take them out of the oven.

19. What is the correct order for adding these ingredients?

   a. Brown sugar, baking soda, chocolate chips
   b. Baking soda, brown sugar, chocolate chips
   c. Chocolate chips, baking soda, brown sugar
   d. Baking soda, chocolate chips, brown sugar

20. What does sturdy mean?

   a. Long
   b. Strong
   c. Short
   d. Wide

21. What does disperse mean?

   a. Scatter
   b. To form a ball
   c. To stir
   d. To beat

22. When can you stop stirring the nuts?

   a. When the cookies are cooked.
   b. When the nuts are evenly distributed.
   c. When the nuts are added.
   d. After the chocolate chips are added.

Questions 23 - 26 refer to the following passage.

Passage 5 - Frankenstein

Great God! What a scene has just taken place! I am yet dizzy with the remembrance of it. I hardly know whether I shall have the power to detail it; yet the tale which I have recorded would be incomplete without this final and wonderful catastrophe. I entered the cabin where lay the remains of my ill-fated and admirable friend. Over him hung a form which I cannot find words to describe—gigantic in stature, yet uncouth and distorted in its proportions. As he hung over the coffin, his face was concealed by long locks of ragged hair; but one vast hand was extended, in color and apparent texture like that of a mummy. When he heard the sound of my approach, he ceased to utter exclamations of grief and horror and sprung towards the window. Never did I behold a vision so horrible as his face, of such loathsome yet appalling hideousness. I shut my eyes involuntarily and endeavored to recollect what were my duties with regard to this destroyer. I called on him to stay.

He paused, looking on me with wonder, and again turning towards the lifeless form of his creator, he seemed to forget my presence, and every feature and gesture seemed instigated by the wildest rage of some uncontrollable passion.

"That is also my victim!" he exclaimed. "In his murder my crimes are consummated; the miserable series of my being is wound to its close! Oh, Frankenstein! Generous and self-devoted being! What does it avail that I now ask thee to pardon me? I, who irretrievably destroyed thee by destroying all thou lovedst. Alas! He is cold, he cannot answer me."

His voice seemed suffocated, and my first impulses, which had suggested to me the duty of obeying the dying request of my friend in destroying his enemy, were now suspended by a mixture of curiosity and compassion. I approached this tremendous being; I dared not again raise my eyes to his face, there was something so scaring and unearthly in his ugliness. I attempted to speak, but the words died away on my lips. The monster continued to utter wild and incoherent self-reproaches. At length I gathered resolution to address him in a pause of the tempest of his passion.

"Your repentance," I said, "is now superfluous. If you had listened to the voice of conscience and heeded the stings of remorse before you had urged your diabolical vengeance to this extremity, Frankenstein would yet have lived." [7]

23. Who is the "ill-fated and admirable friend" who is lying in the coffin?

    a. Frankenstein's monster

    b. Frankenstein

    c. Mary Shelley

    d. Unknown

24. Why is the speaker 'suspended" from following through on his duty to destroy the monster?

    a. The way the monster looks

    b. The monster's remorse

    c. Curiosity and compassion

    d. Fear the monster might kill him too

25. How does Frankenstein's monster destroy Frankenstein?

    a. By killing Frankenstein

    b. By letting himself be the monster everyone sees him as

    c. By destroying everything Frankenstein loved

    d. All of the above

Practice Test Questions Set 2

26. When the Speaker says the monster's repentance is "superfluous," what does he mean?

    a. That it is unnecessary and unused because Frankenstein is already dead and cannot hear him

    b. That he accepts the repentance on behalf of Frankenstein

    c. That the monster does not actually feel remorseful

    d. That his repentance is unneeded because he did not do anything wrong

Questions 27 - 30 refer to the following passage.

Lowest Price Guarantee

Get it for less. Guaranteed!

ABC Electric will beat any advertised price by 10% of the difference.

    1) If you find a lower advertised price, we will beat it by 10% of the difference.

    2) If you find a lower advertised price within 30 days* of your purchase we will beat it by 10% of the difference.

    3) If our own price is reduced within 30 days* of your purchase, bring in your receipt and we will refund the difference.

*14 days for computers, monitors, printers, laptops, tablets, cellular & wireless devices, home security products, projectors, camcorders, digital cameras, radar detectors, portable DVD players, DJ and pro-audio equipment, and air conditioners.

27. I bought a radar detector 15 days ago and saw an ad for the same model only cheaper. Can I get 10% of the difference refunded?

    a. Yes. Since it is less than 30 days, you can get 10% of the difference refunded.

    b. No. Since it is more than 14 days, you cannot get 10% of the difference re-funded.

    c. It depends on the cashier.

    d. Yes. You can get the difference refunded.

28. I bought a flat-screen TV for $500 10 days ago and found an advertisement for the same TV, at another store, on sale for $400. How much will ABC refund under this guarantee?

   a. $100
   b. $110
   c. $10
   d. $400

29. What is the purpose of this passage?

   a. To inform
   b. To educate
   c. To persuade
   d. To entertain

Questions 30 - 33 refer to the following passage.

Passage 6 - What Is Mardi Gras?

Mardi Gras is fast becoming one of the South's most famous and most celebrated holidays. The word Mardi Gras comes from the French and the literal translation is "Fat Tuesday." The holiday has also been called Shrove Tuesday, due to its associations with Lent. The purpose of Mardi Gras is to celebrate and enjoy before the Lenten season of fasting and repentance begins.

What originated by the French Explorers in New Orleans, Louisiana in the 17th century is now celebrated all over the world. Panama, Italy, Belgium and Brazil all host large scale Mardi Gras celebrations, and many smaller cities and towns celebrate this fun loving Tuesday as well. Usually held in February or early March, Mardi Gras is a day of extravagance, a day for people to eat, drink and be merry, to wear costumes, masks and to dance to jazz music.

The French explorers on the Mississippi River would be in shock today if they saw the opulence of the parades and floats that grace the New Orleans streets during Mardi Gras these days. Parades in New Orleans are divided by organizations. These are more commonly known as Krewes.

Being a member of a Krewe is quite a task because Krewes are responsible for overseeing the parades. Each Krewe's parade is ruled by a Mardi Gras "King and Queen." The role of the King and Queen is to "bestow" gifts on their adoring fans as the floats ride along the street. They throw doubloons, which is fake money and usually colored green, purple and gold, which are the colors of Mardi Gras. Beads in those color shades are also thrown and cups are thrown as well. Beads are by far the most popular souvenir of any Mardi Gras parade, with each spectator attempting to gather as many as possible.

30. The purpose of Mardi Gras is to

   a. Repent for a month.

   b. Celebrate in extravagant ways.

   c. Be a member of a Krewe.

   d. Explore the Mississippi.

31. From reading the passage we can infer that "Kings and Queens"

   a. Have to be members of a Krewe.

   b. Have to be French.

   c. Have to know how to speak French.

   d. Have to give away their own money.

32. Which group of people first began to hold Mardi Gras celebrations?

   a. Settlers from Italy

   b. Members of Krewes

   c. French explorers

   d. Belgium explorers

33. In the context of the passage, what does the word spectator most nearly mean?

   a. Someone who participates actively

   b. Someone who watches the parade's action

   c. Someone on one of the parade floats

   d. Someone who does not celebrate Mardi Gras

Questions 34 - 35 refer to the following passage.

Passage 7 - Peter Pan

Author: James M. Barrie

All children, except one, grow up. They soon know that they will grow up, and the way Wendy knew was this. One day when she was two years old she was playing in a garden, and she plucked another flower and ran with it to her mother. I suppose she must have looked rather delightful, for Mrs. Darling put her hand to her heart and cried, "Oh, why can't you remain like this for ever!" This was all that passed between them on the subject, but henceforth Wendy knew that she must grow up. You always know after you are two. Two is the beginning of the end.
Of course they lived at 14 [their house number on their street], and

until Wendy came her mother was the chief one. She was a lovely lady, with a romantic mind and such a sweet mocking mouth. Her romantic mind was like the tiny boxes, one within the other, that come from the puzzling East, however many you discover there is always one more; and her sweet mocking mouth had one kiss on it that Wendy could never get, though there it was, perfectly conspicuous in the right-hand corner.

The way Mr. Darling won her was this: the many gentlemen who had been boys when she was a girl discovered simultaneously that they loved her, and they all ran to her house to propose to her except Mr. Darling, who took a cab and nipped in first, and so he got her. He got all of her, except the innermost box and the kiss. He never knew about the box, and in time he gave up trying for the kiss. Wendy thought Napoleon could have got it, but I can picture him trying, and then going off in a

passion, slamming the door.

34. The author's description of Mrs. Darling's "sweet mocking mouth" implies:

    a. While pretty, Mrs. Darling frequently chides others.

    b. Although subject to slight disfigurement, Mrs. Darling's mouth is still pleasant in appearance.

    c. Mrs. Darling uses her words to get her way.

    d. Mrs. Darling is a loving woman, yet she does not wholly give her love away.

35. Overall, from this passage you can infer that Mrs. Darling:

    a. Is a dominant, complex woman.

    b. Accidentally denies those around her.

    c. Is artistic and absent-minded.

    d. Has a troubled marriage.

Section II – Math

1. Richard gives 's' amount of salary to each of his 'n' employees weekly. If he has 'x' amount of money, how many days he can employ these 'n' employees.

    a. sx/7n
    b. 7x/nx
    c. nx/7s
    d. 7x/ns

2. Translate the following into an equation: Five greater than 3 times a number.

    a. 3X + 5
    b. 5X + 3
    c. (5 + 3)X
    d. 5(3 + X)

3. What number is MMXIII?

    a. 2010
    b. 1990
    c. 2013
    d. 2012

4. Solve for x, when 5x + 21 = 66.

    a. 19
    b. 9
    c. 15
    d. 5

5. Write 765.3682 to the nearest 1000th.

    a. 765.368
    b. 765.36
    c. 765.3682
    d. 765.3

6. If Lynn can type a page in p minutes, what portion of the page can she do in 5 minutes?

    a. p/5
    b. p - 5
    c. p + 5
    d. 5/p

7. If Sally can paint a house in 4 hours, and John can paint the same house in 6 hours, how long will it take for both of to paint a house?

    a. 2 hours and 24 minutes
    b. 3 hours and 12 minutes
    c. 3 hours and 44 minutes
    d. 4 hours and 10 minutes

8. Employees of a discount appliance store receive an additional 20% off the lowest price on any item. If an employee purchases a dishwasher during a 15% off sale, how much will he pay if the dishwasher originally cost $450?

    a. $280.90
    b. $287.00
    c. $292.50
    d. $306.00

9. The sale price of a car is $12,590, which is 20% off the original price. What is the original price?

   a. $14,310.40
   b. $14,990.90
   c. $15,108.00
   d. $15,737.50

10. Express 25% as a fraction.

    a. 1/4
    b. 7/40
    c. 6/25
    d. 8/28

11. Express 125% as a decimal.

    a. .125
    b. 12.5
    c. 1.25
    d. 125

12. Express 24/56 as a reduced common fraction.

    a. 4/9
    b. 4/11
    c. 3/7
    d. 3/8

13. Express 71/1000 as a decimal.

    a. .71
    b. .0071
    c. .071
    d. 7.1

14. What number is in the ten thousandths place in 1.7389?

    a. 1
    b. 8
    c. 9
    d. 3

15. Simplify 6 3/5 − 4 4/5

    a. 1 4/5
    b. 2 3/5
    c. 2 9/5
    d. 1 1/5

16. The physician ordered 100 mg Ibuprofen/kg of body weight; on hand is 230 mg/tablet. The child weighs 50 lb. How many tablets will you give?

    a. 10 tablets
    b. 5 tablets
    c. 1 tablet
    d. 12 tablets

17. In wa local election at polling station A, 945 voters cast their vote out of 1270 registered voters. At polling station B, 860 cast their vote out of 1050 registered voters and at station C, 1210 cast their vote out of 1440 registered voters. What is the total turnout from all three polling stations?

    a. 70%
    b. 74%
    c. 76%
    d. 80%

18. The physician ordered 600 mg ibuprofen; the pharmacy stocks 200 mg per tablet. How many tablets will you give?

   a. 3.5 tablets
   b. 2 tablets
   c. 5 tablets
   d. 3 tablets

19. The manager of a weaving factory estimates that if 10 machines run at 100% efficiency for 8 hours, they will produce 1450 meters of cloth. Due to some technical problems, 4 machines run of 95% efficiency and the remaining 6 at 90% efficiency. How many meters of cloth can these machines will produce in 8 hours?

   a. 1334 meters
   b. 1310 meters
   c. 1300 meters
   d. 1285 meters

20. Convert 60 feet to inches.

   a. 700 inches
   b. 600 inches
   c. 720 inches
   d. 1,800 inches

21. A box contains 7 black pencils and 28 blue ones. What is the ratio between the black and blue pens?

   a. 1:4
   b. 2:7
   c. 1:8
   d. 1:9

22. Convert 100 millimeters to centimeters.

   a. 10 centimeters
   b. 1,000 centimeters
   c. 1100 centimeters
   d. 50 centimeters

23. Convert 3 gallons to quarts.

   a. 15 quarts
   b. 6 quarts
   c. 12 quarts
   d. 32 quarts

24. A map uses a scale of 1:2,000 How much distance on the ground is 5.2 inches on the map if the scale is in inches?

   a. 100,400
   b. 10, 500
   c. 10,440
   d. 10,400

25. 0.05 ml. =

   a. 50 liters
   b. 0.00005 liters
   c. 5 liters
   d. 0.0005 liters

26. X% of 120 = 30. Solve for X.

   a. 15
   b. 12
   c. 4
   d. 25

27. Smith and Simon are playing a card game. Smith will win if a card drawn from a deck of 52 is either 7 or a diamond, and Simon will win if the drawn card is an even number. Which statement is more likely to be correct?

   a. Smith will win more games.
   b. Simon will win more games.
   c. They have same winning probability.
   d. A decision cannot be made from the provided data.

28. Convert .45 meters to centimeters

   a. 45
   b. 450
   c. 4.5
   d. .45

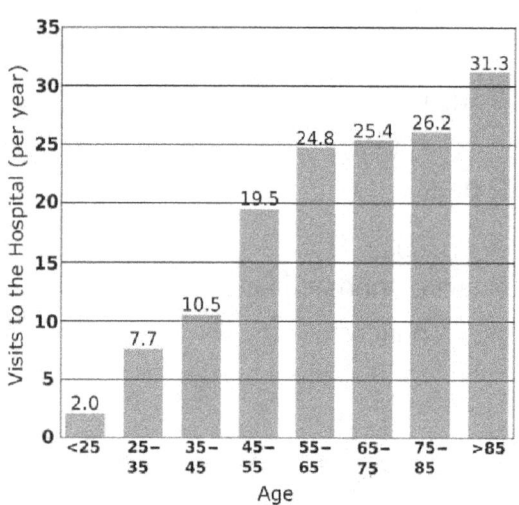

29. Consider the graph above.

How many hospital visits per year does a person aged 85 or more make?

   a. 26.2
   b. 31.3
   c. More than 31.3
   d. A decision cannot be made from this graph.

30. Based on this graph, how many visits per year do you expect a person that is 95 or older to make?

   a. 31.3 or more
   b. Less than 31.3
   c. 31.3
   d. A decision cannot be made from this graph.

Section III – English and Language Usage

1. Elaine promised to bring the camera _____ at the mall yesterday.

   a. by me
   b. with me
   c. at me
   d. to me

2. Last night, he _____ the sleeping bag down beside my mattress.

   a. lay
   b. laid
   c. lain
   d. has laid

3. I would have bought the shirt for you if

   a. I had known you liked it.
   b. I have known you liked it.
   c. I would know you liked it.
   d. I know you liked it.

4. Many believers still hope _____ proof of the existence of ghosts.

    a. two find

    b. to find

    c. to found

    d. to have been found

5. Choose the sentence with the correct grammar.

    a. The court summons was placed on his desk

    b. The court summons are placed on his desk

    c. The court summons were placed on his desk

    d. None of the above

6. To _____, Anne was on time for her math class.

    a. everybody's surprise

    b. every body's surprise

    c. everybodys surprise

    d. everybodys' surprise

7. As an added bonus, we got to see the orchestra warm up.

What part of this sentence is redundant?

    a. Added

    b. Bonus

    c. Warm up

    d. None of the above

8. If he _____ the textbook like he was supposed to, he would have known what was on the test.

    a. will have read

    b. shouldn't have read

    c. would have read

    d. had read

9. Following the tornado, telephone poles _____ all over the street.

   a. laid
   b. lied
   c. were lying
   d. were laying

10. In Edgar Allen Poe's _____ Edgar Allen Poe describes a man with a guilty conscience.

    a. short story, "The Tell-Tale Heart,"
    b. short story The Tell-Tale Heart,
    c. short story, The Tell-Tale Heart
    d. short story. "the Tell-Tale Heart,"

11. Billboards are considered an important part of advertising for big business, _____ by their critics.

    a. but, an eyesore;
    b. but, " an eyesore,"
    c. but an eyesore
    d. but-an eyesore-

12. I can never remember how to use those two common words, "sell," meaning to trade a product for money, or _____ meaning an event where products are traded for less money than usual.

    a. sale-
    b. "sale,"
    c. "sale
    d. "to sale,"

13. Choose the sentence with the correct grammar.

    a. Neither the teacher nor the students is left in class.
    b. Neither the teacher nor the students was left in class.
    c. Neither the teacher nor the students are left in class.
    d. None of the above.

14. **The class just finished reading _____ a short story by Carl Stephenson about a plantation owner's battle with army ants.**

   a. -"Leinengen versus the Ants,"
   b. Leinengen versus the Ants,
   c. "Leinengen versus the Ants,"
   d. Leinengen versus the Ants

15. **After the car was fixed, it _____ again.**

   a. ran good
   b. ran well
   c. would have run well
   d. ran more well

16. **"Where does the sun go during the _____ asked little Kathy.**

   a. night,"
   b. night"?,
   c. night,?"
   d. night?"

17. **Choose the correct spelling.**

   a. conscentious
   b. conscientios
   c. conscientious
   d. consceintious

18. **I have finished studying for today.**

What type of sentence is this?

   a. Imperative
   b. Interrogative
   c. Exclamatory
   d. Declarative

19. Which of the following sentences contains a redundant phrase?

a. I haven't seen her for ages.
b. My suitcase is books all the way to Amsterdam.
c. The end result was very disappointing.
d. None of the above.

20. Choose the correct sentence.

a. Their only employee with a nose ring is a young man named Daniel.
b. Their only employee is a young man named Daniel with a nose ring.
c. Their only employee is a young man with a nose ring named Daniel.
d. A and C are correct.

21. Choose the sentence with the correct grammar.

a. Everyone are to wear a black tie.
b. Everyone have to wear a black tie.
c. Everyone has to wear a black tie.
d. None of the above.

22. Choose the correct spelling.

a. leisuire
b. lesure
c. lesure
d. leisure

23. Choose the correct spelling.

a. pigeone
b. pigoen
c. pigeon
d. pidgeon

24. Choose the correct spelling.

a. odyessy
b. odeyssey
c. odysey
d. odyssey

25. Choose the sentence with the correct grammar.

    a. The salmon has been cooked.
    b. The salmon have been cooked.
    c. Both of the above.
    d. None of the above.

26. This is absolutely incredible ____

    a. !
    b. .
    c. :
    d. ;

27. Watch out for the broken glass ____

    a. .
    b. ?
    c. ,
    d. !

28. I still don't know exactly. That isn't _____ evidence.

    a. Undeterred
    b. Unrelenting
    c. Unfortunate
    d. Conclusive

29. He walked all the way downtown.

What is the simple subject of this sentence?

    a. He
    b. Walked
    c. Downtown
    d. All the way

30. He could manipulate the coins in his fingers very

   a. Brazenly
   b. Eloquently
   c. Boisterously
   d. Deftly

Section IV – Science

1. Which of the following is not true

   a. Genotypes are inherited information
   b. Phenotypes are inherited information
   c. Phenotypes are observed behavior
   d. Phenotypes include an organisms development

2. Electrons play a critical role in

   a. Electricity
   b. Magnetism
   c. Thermal conductivity
   d. All of the above

3. An idea concerning a phenomena and possible explanations for that phenomena is a/an

   a. Theory
   b. Experiment
   c. Inference
   d. Hypothesis

4. Define chromosomes.

   a. Structures in a cell nucleus that carry genetic material.
   b. Consist of thousands of DNA strands.
   c. Total 46 in a normal human cell.
   d. All of the above

5. What is one of the best known disorders that attack the immune system?

   a. Rabies

   b. HIV

   c. Lung cancer

   d. Muscular dystrophy

6. Which disease of the circulatory system is one of the most frequent causes of death in North America?

   a. The cold

   b. Pneumonia

   c. Arthritis

   d. Heart disease

7. Which of the following describes a plasma membrane?

   a. Lipids with embedded proteins

   b. An outer lipid layer and an inner lipid layer

   c. Proteins embedded in lipid bilayer

   d. Altering protein and lipid layers

8. What is the difference between Strong Nuclear Force and Weak Nuclear Force?

   a. The Strong Nuclear Force is an attractive force that binds protons and neutrons and maintains the structure of the nucleus, and the Weak Nuclear Force is responsible for the radioactive beta decay and other subatomic reactions.

   b. The Strong Nuclear Force is responsible for the radioactive beta decay and other subatomic reactions, and the Weak Nuclear Force is an attractive force that binds protons and neutrons and maintains the structure of the nucleus.

   c. The Weak Nuclear Force is feeble and the Strong Nuclear Force is robust.

   d. The Strong Nuclear Force is a negative force that releases protons and neutrons and threatens the structure of the nucleus, and the Weak Nuclear Force is an attractive force that binds protons and neutrons and maintains the structure of the nucleus.

9. What type of research studies the quality, type or components of a group, substance, or mixture?

   a. Quantitative

   b. Dependent

   c. Scientific

   d. Qualitative

10. Adaptation is

a. A trait that has evolved by natural selection.

b. A trait that has been bred by artificial selection.

c. A trait that has no function in an organism.

d. None of the above.

11. Describe a pH indicator.

a. A pH indicator measures hydrogen ions in a solution and show pH on a color scale.

b. A pH indicator measures oxygen ions in a solution and show pH on a color scale.

c. A pH indicator many different types of ions in a solution and shows pH on a color scale.

d. None of the above.

12. What is the earth's primary source of energy?

a. Water

b. The sun

c. Electromagnetic radiation

d. Weak nuclear force

13. What type of research is to determine the relationship between one thing (an independent variable) and another (a dependent or outcome variable) in a population?

a. Qualitative

b. Quantitative

c. Independent

d. Scientific

14. What can accept a hydrogen ion and can react with fats to form soaps?

a. Acid

b. Salt

c. Base

d. Foundation

Practice Test Questions Set 2

15. Which gene, whose presence as a single copy, controls the expression of a trait?

   a. Principal gene
   b. Latent gene
   c. Recessive gene
   d. Dominant gene

16. Within taxonomy, plants and animals are considered two basic

   a. Families
   b. Kingdoms
   c. Domains
   d. Genus

17. Organisms grouped into the _____ Kingdom include all unicellular organisms lacking a definite cellular arrangement such as _____ and _____.

   a. Fungi, bacteria, algae
   b. Protista, bacteria, amphibian
   c. Protista, bacteria, algae
   d. Plantae, bacteria, algae

18. What is a common digestive affliction most people suffer at one time or other?

   a. Stomach cancer
   b. Ulceritis
   c. Indigestion
   d. The flu

19. What are the biochemical and biophysical activities that all living systems must be able to carry out to maintain life?

   a. Life sequences
   b. Life expectancies
   c. Life cycles
   d. Life functions

20. **What disease of the circulatory system is often mistaken for a heart attack?**

   a. Cardiac arrest
   b. High blood pressure
   c. Angina
   d. Acid reflux

21. **Define a biological class.**

   a. A collection of similar or like living entities.
   b. Two or more animals in a group, all having the same parent.
   c. All animals sharing the same living environment.
   d. All plant life that share the same physical properties.

22. **What type of foods that stay in the stomach the longest?**

   a. Fats
   b. Proteins
   c. Carbohydrates
   d. Vitamins

23. **What is a graphical description of feeding relationships among species in an ecological community?**

   a. Food web
   b. Food chain
   c. Food network
   d. Food sequence

24. **What is the diagram that is used to predict an outcome of a particular cross or breeding experiment?**

   a. Genetic puzzle
   b. Genome project
   c. Hybrid theorem
   d. Punnett square

Practice Test Questions Set 2

25. Which, if any, of the following statements about prokaryotic cells is false?

    a. Prokaryotic cells include such organisms as E. coli and Streptococcus.
    b. Prokaryotic cells lack internal membranes and organelles.
    c. Prokaryotic cells break down food using cellular respiration and fermentation.
    d. All of these statements are true.

26. What is the process of converting observed phenomena into data is called?

    a. Calculation
    b. Measurement
    c. Valuation
    d. Estimation

27. The mass number of an atom is

    a. The total number of particles that make it up.
    b. The total weight of an atom.
    c. The total mass of an atom.
    d. None of the above.

28. What is sublimation?

    a. A phase transition from liquid to gas.
    b. A phase transition from solid to gas.
    c. A phase transition from gas to liquid.
    d. A phase transition from gas to solid.

29. How is exhalation accomplished?

    a. By the abdominal muscles
    b. By the chest muscles
    c. By the esophagus
    d. By the nasal passageway

30. What three processes are involved in cell division of Eukaryotic cells?

    a. Meiosis, mitosis, and interphase
    b. Meiosis, mitosis, and interphase
    c. Mitosis, kinematisis, and interphase
    d. Mitosis, cytokinesis, and interphase

31. **Describe genotypes.**

    a. The genetic makeup, as distinguished from the physical appearance, of an organism or a group of organisms.

    b. The combination of alleles located on homologous chromosomes that determines a specific characteristic or trait.

    c. Is the inheritable information carried by all living organisms.

    d. All of the above.

32. **What does the respiratory system primarily oxygenate?**

    a. The brain
    b. The limbs
    c. The heart
    d. The blood

33. **What chain of nucleotides plays an important role in the creation of new proteins?**

    a. Deoxyribonucleic acid (DNA) is a chain of nucleotides that plays an important role in the creation of new proteins.

    b. Ribonucleic acid (RNA) is a chain of nucleotides that plays an important role in the creation of new proteins.

    c. There are no chains of nucleotides that play a role in the creation of proteins.

    d. None of the above.

34. **A practical test designed with the intention that its results will be relevant to a particular theory or set of theories is a/an**

    a. Experiment
    b. Practicum
    c. Theory
    d. Design

35. **Strong chemical bonds include**

    a. Dipole - dipole interactions.
    b. Hydrogen bonding.
    c. Covalent or ionic bonds.
    d. None of the above.

Practice Test Questions Set 2

36. What is the process that the immune system adapts over time to be more efficient in recognizing pathogens?

    a. Acquired immunity

    b. AIDS

    c. Pathogens

    d. Acquired deficiency

37. What is a group of tissues that perform a specific function or group of functions?

    a. System

    b. Tissue

    c. Group

    d. Organ

38. What is the measure of an experiment's ability to yield the same or compatible results in different clinical experiments or statistical trials?

    a. Variability

    b. Validity

    c. Control measure

    d. Reliability

39. Describe each chemical element in the periodic table.

    a. Each chemical element has a unique atomic number representing the number of electrons in its nucleus.

    b. Each chemical element has a varying atomic number depending on the number of protons in its nucleus.

    c. Each chemical element has a unique atomic number representing the number of protons in its nucleus.

    d. None of the above.

40. The immune system is

    a. The system that expels waste from the body.

    b. The system that expels carbon dioxide from the body.

    c. The system that protects the body from disease and infection.

    d. The system that circulates blood through the body.

41. The binding membrane of an animal cell is called

    a. The biological membrane.

    b. The cell coat.

    c. The unit membrane.

    d. The plasma membrane.

42. Define organelles.

    a. A protein in a cell

    b. An enzyme in a cell

    c. A specialized subunit of a cell with a specific function

    d. A cell membrane

43. A solution with a pH value of less than 7 is

    a. Acid solution.

    b. Base solution.

    c. Neutral pH solution.

    d. None of the above.

44. Is a catalyst changed by a reaction?

    a. Yes

    b. No

    c. It may be changed depending on the other chemicals.

45. What is the prediction that an observed difference is due to chance alone and not due to a systematic cause? This hypothesis is tested by statistical analysis, and either accepted or rejected.

    a. Null hypothesis

    b. Hypothesis

    c. Control

    d. Variable

46. In science, industry, and statistics, the _____ of a measurement system is the degree of closeness of measurements of a quantity to its actual (true) value.

   a. Mistake
   b. Uncertainty
   c. Accuracy
   d. Error

47. What is a more common name for the circulatory system disease known as hypertension?

   a. Anemia
   b. High blood pressure
   c. Angina
   d. Cardiac arrest

48. Given a normal distribution, what is the difference between the maximum value and the minimum value?

   a. Distribution
   b. Range
   c. Mode
   d. Median

Quick Reference Answer Key

Part I - Reading

1. A
2. C
3. D
4. A
5. B
6. C
7. B
8. A
9. D
10. B
11. A
12. A
13. C
14. C
15. A
16. B
17. A
18. B
19. A
20. B
21. A
22. B
23. B
24. C
25. D
26. A
27. B
28. B
29. C
30. B
31. A
32. C
33. B
34. D
35. A

Section II – Math

1. D
2. A
3. C
4. B
5. A
6. D
7. A
8. D
9. D
10. A
11. C
12. C
13. C
14. C
15. A
16. A
17. D
18. D
19. A
20. C
21. A
22. A
23. C
24. D
25. B
26. D
27. B
28. A
29. A
30. A

Section III – English and Language Usage

1. D
2. A
3. A
4. B
5. A
6. A
7. A
8. D
9. C
10. A
11. C
12. B
13. C
14. C
15. B

16. D
17. C
18. D
19. C
20. D
21. C
22. D
23. C
24. D
25. C
26. A
27. D
28. D
29. A
30. D

30. D
31. D
32. D
33. B
34. A
35. C
36. A
37. D
38. D
39. C
40. C
41. D
42. C
43. A
44. B
45. A
46. C
47. B
48. B

Section IV – Science

1. B
2. D
3. D
4. D
5. B
6. D
7. C
8. A
9. D
10. A
11. A
12. B
13. B
14. C
15. D
16. B
17. C
18. C
19. D
20. C
21. A
22. A
23. A
24. D
25. D
26. B
27. A
28. B
29. A

Answer Key with Explanations

1. A

Choice B is incorrect; the author did not express their opinion on the subject matter. Choice C is incorrect, the author was not trying to prove a point.

2. C

Choice C is correct; historians believe it was brutal and bloody. Choice A is incorrect; there is no consensus that the Crusades achieved great things. Choice B is incorrect; it did not stabilize the Holy Lands. Choice D is incorrect, some historians do believe this was the purpose but not all historians.

3. D

The feudal system led to infighting. Choice A is incorrect, it had the opposite effect. Choice B is incorrect, though this is a good answer, it is not the best answer. The Church asked for volunteers not the Feudal Lords. Choice C is incorrect, it did have an effect on the Crusades.

4. A

Saracen was a generic term for Muslims widely used in Europe during the later medieval era.

5. B

This warranty does not cover a product that you have tried to fix yourself. From paragraph two, "This limited warranty does not cover ... any unauthorized disassembly, repair, or modification. "

6. C

ABC Electric could either replace or repair the fan, provided the other conditions are met. ABC Electric has the option to repair or replace.

7. B

The warranty does not cover a stove damaged in a flood. From the passage, "This limited warranty does not cover any damage to the product from improper installation, accident, abuse, misuse, natural disaster, insufficient or excessive electrical supply, abnormal mechanical or environmental conditions."

A flood is an "abnormal environmental condition," and a natural disaster, so it is not covered.

8. A

A missing part is an example of defective workmanship. This is an error made in the manufacturing process. A defective part is not considered workmanship.

9. D

This question tests the reader's summarization skills. The other choices A, B, and C focus on portions of the second paragraph that are too narrow and do not relate to the specific portion of text in question. The complexity of the sentence may mislead students into selecting one of these answers, but rearranging or restating the sentence will lead the reader to the correct answer. In addition, choice A makes an assumption that may or may not be true about the intentions of the company, choice B focuses on one product rather than the idea of the products, and choice C makes an assumption about women that may or may not be true and is not supported by the text.

10. B
This question tests reader's attention to detail. If a reader selects A, he or she may have picked up on the use of the word "debate" and assumed, very logically, that the two are at odds because they are fighting; however, this is simply not supported in the text. Choice C also uses very specific quotes from the text, but it rearranges and gives them false meaning. The artists want to elevate their creations above the creations of other artists, thereby showing that they are "creative" and "innovative." Similarly, choice D takes phrases straight from the text and rearranges and confuses them. The artists are described as wanting to be "creative, innovative, individual people," not the women.

11. A
This question tests reader's vocabulary and summarization skills. This phrase, used by the author, may seem flippant and dismissive if readers focus on the word "whatever" and misinterpret it as a popular, colloquial term. In this way, choices B and C may mislead the reader to selecting one of them by including the terms "unimportant" and "stupid," respectively. Choice D is a similar misreading, but doesn't make sense when the phrase is at the beginning of the passage and the entire passage is on media messages. Choice A is literally and contextually appropriate, and the reader can understand that the author would like to keep the introduction focused on the topic the passage is going to discuss.

12. A
This question tests a reader's inference skills. The extreme use of the word "all" in choice B suggests that every single advertising company are working to be approachable, and while this is not only unlikely, the text specifically states that "more" companies have done this, signifying that they have not all participated, even if it's a possibility that they may some day. The use of the limiting word "only" in choice C lends that answer similar problems; women are still buying from companies who do not care about this message, or those companies would not be in business, and the passage specifies that "many" women are worried about media messages, but not all. Readers may find choice D logical, especially if they are looking to make an inference, and while this may be a possibility, the passage does not suggest or discuss this happening. Choice A is correct based on specifically because of the relation between "still working" in the answer and "will hopefully" and the extensive discussion on companies struggles, which come only with progress, in the text.

13. C
This question tests the reader's summarization skills. The entire passage is leading up to the idea that the president of the US may not have had grounds to assert his Fourteen Points when other countries had lost so much. Choice A is pretty directly inferred by the text, but it does not adequately summarize what the entire passage is trying to communicate. Choice B may also be inferred by the passage when it says that the war is "imminent," but it does not represent the entire message, either. The passage does seem to be in praise of FDR, or at least in respect of him, but it does not in any way

claim that he is the smartest president, nor does this represent the many other points included. Choice C is then the obvious answer, and most directly relates to the closing sentences which it rewords.

14. C
This question tests the reader's attention to detail. The passage does state that choices A and B are true, and while those statements are in proximity to the explanation for why the war started, they are not the reason given. Choice D is a mix up of words used in the passage, which says that the largest powers were in play but not that this fact somehow started the war. The passage does make a direct statement that a domino effect started the war, supporting choice C as the correct answer.

15. A
This question tests the reader's understanding of functions in writing. Throughout the passage, it states that leaders of other nations were hesitant to accept generous or peaceful terms because of the grievances of the war, and the great loss of life was chief among these. While the passage does touch on the devastation of deadly weapons (B), the use of this raw, emotional fact serves a much larger purpose, and the focus of the passage is not the weapons. While readers may indeed consider who lost the most soldiers (C) when, so many countries were involved and the inequalities of loss are mentioned in the passage, there is no discussion of this in the passage. Choice D is related to A, but choice A is more direct and relates more to the passage.

16. B
This question tests the reader's vocabulary skills. Choice A may seem appealing to readers because it is phonetically similar to "catalyzed," but the two are not related in any other way. Choice C makes sense in context, but if plugged in to the sentence creates a redundancy that doesn't make sense. Choice D does also not make sense contextually, even if the reader may consider that funds were needed to create more weaponry, especially if it was advanced.

17. A
Victoria is about 5 miles from Burnaby.

18. B
The Village Hall is about 5 miles from Victoria.

19. A
The correct order of ingredients is brown sugar, baking soda and chocolate chips.

20. B
Sturdy: strong, solid in structure or person. In context, Stir in chocolate chips by hand with a *sturdy* wooden spoon.

21. A
Disperse: to scatter in different directions or break up. In context, Stir until the chocolate chips and nuts are evenly *dispersed*.

Practice Test Questions Set 2

22. B
You can stop stirring the nuts when they are evenly distributed. From the passage, "Stir until the chocolate chips and nuts are evenly dispersed."

23. B
Choice A is incorrect as the Monster killed Frankenstein, not the other way around. Choice B is correct, Frankenstein is dead. Choice C is incorrect - Mary Shelley is the author. Choice D is incorrect, the person is called Frankenstein.

24. C
The speaker 'suspended' from following through on his duty to destroy the monster due to curiosity and compassion. The other choices may seem reasonable, but are not explicitly given in the passage.

25. D
All the choices are correct. Frankenstein's monster destroys Frankenstein by

    a. By killing Frankenstein
    b. By letting himself be the monster everyone sees him as
    c. By destroying everything Frankenstein loved

26. A
Superfluous means unnecessary. Looking at the context of the word as it is used in the passage:

"Your repentance," I said, "is now superfluous. If you had listened to the voice of conscience and heeded the stings of remorse before you had urged your diabolical vengeance to this extremity, Frankenstein would yet have lived."

27. B
The time limit for radar detectors is 14 days. Since you made the purchase 15 days ago, you do not qualify for the guarantee.

28. B
Since you made the purchase 10 days ago, you are covered by the guarantee. Since it is an advertised price at a different store, ABC Electric will "beat" the price by 10% of the difference, which is,

500 – 400 = 100 – difference in price

100 X 10% = $10 – 10% of the difference

The advertised lower price is $400. ABC will beat this price by 10% so they will refund $100 + 10 = $110.

29. C
The purpose of this passage is to persuade.

30. B
The correct answer can be found in the fourth sentence of the first paragraph.

Choice A is incorrect because repenting begins the day AFTER Mardi Gras. Choice C is incorrect because you can celebrate Mardi Gras without being a member of a Krewe.

Choice D is incorrect because exploration does not play any role in a modern Mardi Gras celebration.

31. A
The second sentence is the last paragraph states that Krewes are led by the Kings and Queens. Therefore, you must have to be part of a Krewe to be its King or its Queen.

Choice B is incorrect because it never states in the passage that only people from France can be Kings and Queen of Mardi Gras

Choice C is incorrect because the passage says nothing about having to speak French.

Choice D is incorrect because the passage does state that the Kings and Queens throw doubloons, which is fake money.

32. C
The first sentences of BOTH the 2nd and 3rd paragraphs mention that French explorers started this tradition in New Orleans.
Choices A, B and D are incorrect because they are just names of cities or countries listed in the 2nd paragraph.

33. B
In the final paragraph the word spectator is used to describe people who are watching the parade and catching cups, beads and doubloons.
Choices A and C are incorrect because we know the people who participate are part of Krewes. People who work the floats and parades are also part of Krewes

Choice D is incorrect because the passage makes no mention of people who do not celebrate Mardi Gras.

34. D
There is no concrete evidence of choices A, B, or C. Choice D is therefore the best answer, and the passage supports the notion that her mouth possess a special kiss that neither her daughter nor husband can attain, and in this way her mouth seems to mock them.

35. A
Choice A is the best-supported choice: The narrator notes, "Until Wendy came, her mother was the chief one," and further describes Mrs. Darling as a woman who will not compromise. Both Mr. Darling and Wendy are seemingly unable to access the full extent of Mrs. Darling's affection. The description of Mrs. Darling's mind as "like the tiny boxes, one within the other, that come from the puzzling East" suggests she is a woman with many layers, is impossible to fully understand, and to this end has even a foreign quality to her. B is incorrect as nothing about her denial of her husband or daughter

appears to be accidental. Choice C's "absent-minded" descriptor could be reasonable, yet "romantic" is not in this case the same as "artistic", and there is no evidence of Mrs. Darling's artistic ability. Again, in light of Mr. Darling giving up on the elusive kiss, choice D could be reasonable, however there is nothing to suggest a serious problem is present in the matrimony. Nothing suggests Mrs. Darling is indecisive, choice E is incorrect.

Section II – Math

1. D
We understand that each of the n employees earn s amount of salary weekly. This means that one employee earns s salary weekly. So; Richard has ns amount of money to employ n employees for a week.

We are asked to find the number of days n employees can be employed with x amount of money. We can do simple direct proportion:

If Richard can employ n employees for 7 days with ns amount of money,

Richard can employ n employees for y days with x amount of money ... y is the number of days we need to find.

We can do cross multiplication:

$y = (x \cdot 7)/(ns)$

$y = 7x/ns$

2. A
Five greater than 3 times a number.
5 + 3 times a number.
3X + 5

3. C
MMXIII is 2013. 1,000 + 1,000 + 10 + 1 + 1 + 1.

4. B
5b + 21 = 66, 5b = 66 − 21 = 45, 5b = 45, b = 45/5 = 9

5. A
The number is 51.738. The last digit, in the 1,000th place, 2, is less than 5, so it is discarded. Answer = 765.368.

6. D
This is a simple direct proportion problem:
If Lynn can type 1 page in p minutes,

she can type x pages in 5 minutes

We do cross multiplication: x•p = 5•1

Then,

x = 5/p

7. A

This is an inverse ration problem.

1/x = 1/a + 1/b where a is the time Sally can paint a house, b is the time John can paint a house, x is the time Sally and John can together paint a house.

So,

1/x = 1/4 + 1/6 ... We use the least common multiple in the denominator that is 24:

1/x = 6/24 + 4/24

1/x = 10/24

x = 24/10

x = 2.4 hours.

In other words; 2 hours + 0.4 hours = 2 hours + 0.4•60 minutes

= 2 hours 24 minutes

8. D
The cost of the dishwasher = $450

15% discount amount = 450•15/100 = $67.5

The discounted price = 450 – 67.5 = $382.5

20% additional discount amount on lowest price = 382.5•20/100 = $76.5

So, the final discounted price = 382.5 - 76.5 = $306.00

9. D
Original price = x,
80/100 = 12590/X,
80X = 1259000,
X = 15,737.50.

10. A
25% = 25/100 = 1/4

11. C
125/100 = 1.25

Practice Test Questions Set 2

12. C
24/56 = 3/7 (divide numerator and denominator by 8)

13. C
Converting a fraction into a decimal – divide the numerator by the denominator – so 71/1000 = .071. Dividing by 1000 moves the decimal point 3 places to the left.

14. C
9 is in the ten thousandths place in 1.7389, which is 4 places to the right of the decimal point.

15. A
(6-4) (3/5 – 4/5) = 2 (3-4/5) = since 3 is less than 4, we would have to subtract 1 from the whole number besides the fraction, therefore 1 4/5

16. A
Step 1: Set up the formula to calculate the dose to be given in mg as per weight of the child:-
Dose ordered X Weight in Kg = Dose to be given
Step 2: 100 mg X 23 kg = 2300 mg
(Convert 50 lb to Kg, 1 lb = 0.4536 kg, hence 50 lb = 50 X 0.4536 = 22.68 kg approx. 23 kg)
2300 mg/230 mg X 1 tablet/1 = 2300/230 = 10 tablets

17. D
To find the total turnout in all three polling stations, we need to proportion the number of voters to the number of all registered voters.

Number of total voters = 945 + 860 + 1210 = 3015

Number of total registered voters = 1270 + 1050 + 1440 = 3760

Percentage turnout over all three polling stations = 3015•100/3760 = 80.19%

Checking the answers, we round 80.19 to the nearest whole number: 80%

18. D
600 mg/ 200 mg X 1 tablet/1 = 600/200 = 3 tablets

19. A
At 100% efficiency 1 machine produces 1450/10 = 145 m of cloth.

At 95% efficiency, 4 machines produce 4•145•95/100 = 551 m of cloth.

At 90% efficiency, 6 machines produce 6•145•90/100 = 783 m of cloth.

Total cloth produced by all 10 machines = 551 + 783 = 1334 m

Since the information provided and the question are based on 8 hours, we did not need to use time to reach the answer.

20. C

1 foot = 12 inches, 60 feet = 60 x 12 = 720 inches.

21. A

The ratio between black and blue pens is 7 to 28 or 7:28. Bring to the lowest terms by dividing both sides by 7 gives 1:4.

22. A

1 millimeter = 10 centimeter, 100 millimeter = 100/10 = 10 centimeters.

23. C

1 gallon = 4 quarts, 3 gallons = 3 x 4 = 12 quarts.

24. D

1 inch on map = 2,000 inches on ground. So, 5.2 inches on map = 5.2•2,000 = 10,400 inches on ground.

25. B

There are 1000 ml in a liter. 0.05/1000 = 0.00005 liters.

26. D

X% of 120 = 30,
X/100 = 30/120
So X = 30/120 x 100/1
3000/120 = 300/12
X = 25

27. B

There are 52 cards in total. Smith has 16 cards in which he can win. Therefore, his probability of winning in a single game will be 16/52. Simon has 20 winning cards so his probability of winning in single draw is 20/52.

28. A

There are 100 centimeters in a meter, so 100 X .45 meters = 45.

29. A

Based on this graph, a person that is 85 or older will make 26.2 visits to the hospital every year.

30. A

A person aged 95 or older would make 31.3 or more visits.

Section III – English and Language Usage

1. D
The preposition "to" is correct. 'To' here means give.

2. A
"Lie" means to recline, and does not take an object. "lay" means to place and does take an object.

3. A
Past unreal conditional. Takes the form,
[If ... Past Perfect ..., ... would have + past participle ...]

4. B
This sentence is in the present tense, so "to find" is correct.

5. A
Always use the singular verb form for nouns like politics, wages, mathematics, innings, news, advice, summons, furniture, information, poetry, machinery, vacation, scenery etc.

6. A
Possessive pronouns ending in 's' take an apostrophe before the 's': one's; everyone's; somebody's, nobody else's, etc.

7. A
A bonus is an extra feature, so added is redundant.

8. D
When talking about something that didn't happen in the past, use the past perfect (if I had done).

9. C
"Lie" means to recline, and does not take an object. "Lay" means to place and does take an object. Peter lay the books on the table (the books are the direct object), or the telephone poles were lying on the road (no direct object).

10. A
Titles of short stories are enclosed in quotation marks.

11. C
No additional punctuation is required here.

12. B
Here the word "sale" is used as a "word" and not as a word in the sentence, so quotation marks are used.

13. C
If one of the subjects linked by "either," "or," "nor" or "neither" is in plural form, then the verb should also be in plural, and the verb should be close to the plural subject.

14. C
Titles of short stories are enclosed in quotation marks, and commas always go inside quotation marks.

15. B
"Ran well" is correct. "Ran good" is never correct.

16. D
Commas and periods always go inside quotation marks. Question marks that are part of a quote also go inside quotation marks; however, if the writer quotes a statement as part of a larger question, the question mark is placed after the quotation mark.

17. C
Conscientious is the correct spelling.

18. D
This is a declarative sentence.

19. C
A result is something that occurs at the end, so an 'end result' is redundant.

20. D
Both A and C are correct.

   a. Their only employee with a nose ring is a young man named Daniel.
   c. Their only employee is a young man with a nose ring named Daniel.

21. C
Use a singular verb with either, each, neither, everyone and many.

22. D
Leisure is the correct spelling.

23. C
Pigeon is the correct spelling.

24. D
Odyssey is the correct spelling.

25. C
Nouns like deer, sheep, swine, salmon etc can take a singular or plural verb depending if they are used in their singular or plural form.

26. A
Use an exclamation mark to end an exclamatory sentence, that is, at the end of a statement showing strong emotion.

27. D
Use an exclamation mark after an imperative sentence if the command is urgent and forceful.

28. D
Conclusive ADJECTIVE providing an end to something; decisive.

29. A
'He' is the simple subject of this sentence.

30. D
Deftly: VERB. Quick and skillful.

Section IV – Science

1. B
The only statement that is NOT true is, Phenotypes are inherited information.

2. D
All the above are true. Electrons play an essential role in electricity, magnetism, and thermal conductivity.

3. D
An idea concerning a phenomena and possible explanations for that phenomena is an hypothesis.

4. D
All of the above
a. Structures in a cell nucleus that carry genetic material.
b. Consist of one very long strand of DNA
c. Total 46 in a normal human cell.

5. B
One of the best known disorders that attack the immune system is HIV (the virus that causes AIDS).

6. D
The circulatory system disease that is one of the most frequent causes of death in North America is heart disease.

7. C
The plasma membrane or cell membrane protects the cell from outside forces. It consists of the lipid bilayer with embedded proteins.

8. A
The Strong Nuclear Force is an attractive force that binds protons and neutrons and maintains the structure of the nucleus, and the Weak Nuclear Force is responsible for the radioactive beta decay and other subatomic reactions.

9. D
Qualitative research deals with the quality, type or components of a group, substance, or mixture.

10. A
Adaptation is a trait that has evolved by natural selection.

11. A
A pH indicator measures hydrogen ions in a solution and show pH on a color scale.

12. B
The sun is the earth's primary source of energy.

13. B
The goal of quantitative research is to determine the relationship between one thing (an independent variable) and another (a dependent or outcome variable) in a population.

14. C
A base is any substance that can accept a hydrogen ion and can react with fats to form soaps.

15. D
The dominant gene controls the expression of a trait.

16. B
Plants and animals are Kingdoms. There are six recognized kingdoms: Animalia, Plantae, Protista, Fungi, Bacteria, and Archaea.

17. C
Organisms grouped into the **Protista** Kingdom include all unicellular organisms lacking a definite cellular arrangement such as **bacteria** and **algae.**

18. C
Indigestion is a common digestive affliction that most people suffer at one time or other.

19. D
Life functions are the biochemical and biophysical activities that all living systems must be able to carry out to maintain life.

20. C
Angina is frequently mistaken for a heart attack. Angina pectoris, commonly known as angina, is severe chest pain due to ischemia (a lack of blood, thus a lack of oxygen supply) of the heart muscle, generally due to obstruction or spasm of the coronary arteries (the heart's blood vessels). [24]

21. A
A collection of similar or like living entities. Class has the same meaning in biology as

rank. Common classes or ranks include species, order, and phylum.

22. A
Fats stay in the stomach the longest.

23. A
A food web is a graphical description of feeding relationships among species in an ecological community.

Note: A food web differs from a food chain in that the latter shows only a portion of the food web involving a simple, linear series of species (e.g., predator, herbivore, plant) connected by feeding links. A food web aims to depict a more complete picture of the feeding relationships, and can be considered a bundle of many interconnected food chains occurring within the community.

24. D
A Punnett square resembles a game of tic-tac-toe, in which the genotypes of the parents gametes are entered first, so that subsequent combinations can be calculated.

25. D
All of these statements are true.

   a. Prokaryotic cells include such organisms as E. coli and Streptococcus.

   b. Prokaryotic cells lack internal membranes and organelles.

   c. Prokaryotic cells break down food using cellular respiration and fermentation.

26. B
The process of converting observed phenomena into data is called Measurement.

27. A
The mass number of an atom is the total number of particles (protons and neutrons) that make it up.

28. B
Sublimation is the direct phase transition from solid to gas.

29. A
Exhalation is often accomplished by the abdominal muscles.

30. D
In Eukaryotic cells, the cell cycle is the cycle of events involving cell division, including mitosis, cytokinesis, and interphase.

31. D
All of the choices are correct.

   a. The genetic makeup, as distinguished from the physical appearance, of an organism or a group of organisms.

b. The combination of alleles located on homologous chromosomes that determines a specific characteristic or trait.

c. Is the inheritable information carried by all living organisms.

32. D
The blood is the primarily oxygenated through the work of the respiratory system.

33. B
Ribonucleic acid (RNA) is a chain of nucleotides that play an important role in the creation of new proteins.

34. A
A practical test designed with the intention that its results will be relevant to a particular theory or set of theories is an experiment.

35. C
Covalent or ionic bonds are considered "strong bonds."

36. A
The process by which the immune system adapts over time to be more efficient in recognizing pathogens is known as acquired immunity.

37. D
An organ is a group of tissues that perform a specific function or group of functions.

38. D
Reliability refers to the measure of an experiment's ability to yield the same or compatible results in different clinical experiments or statistical trials.

39. C
Each chemical element has a unique atomic number representing the number of protons in its nucleus.

40. C
The immune system is the system that protects the body from disease and infection.

41. D
The plasma membrane surrounds the cell and functions as an interface between the living interior of the cell and the nonliving exterior. [19]

42. C
An organelle is a specialized subunit of a cell with a specific function.

43. A
A solution with a pH value of less than 7 is acid. A pH value of 7 is neutral.

44. B

A catalyst is never changed in a chemical reaction.

45. A

The prediction that an observed difference is due to chance alone and not due to a systematic cause; statistical analysis tested this hypothesis, and it is accepted or rejected is the **null hypothesis**.

46. C

In science and engineering, the Accuracy of a measurement system is the degree of closeness of measurements of a quantity to its actual (true) value.

47. B

High blood pressure is a more common name for the circulatory system disease known as hypertension. Hypertension (HTN) or high blood pressure is a cardiac chronic medical condition in which the systemic arterial blood pressure is elevated.

48. B

The range of a distribution is the difference between the maximum value and the minimum value.

Conclusion

CONGRATULATIONS! You have made it this far because you have applied yourself diligently to practicing for the exam and no doubt improved your potential score considerably! Getting into a good school is a huge step in a journey that might be challenging at times but will be many times more rewarding and fulfilling. That is why being prepared is so important.

Study, then Practice, and then Succeed!

Good Luck!

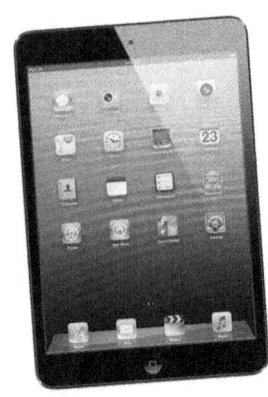

FREE Ebook Version

Go to http://tinyurl.com/m4abcfa

Visit us Online

www.test-preparation.ca

www.study-skills.ca

www.ingramcontent.com/pod-product-compliance
Lightning Source LLC
Chambersburg PA
CBHW080036100526
44584CB00023BA/3227